SICK
and
TIRED

SICK
and
TIRED

How America's Health Care System Fails Its Patients

HELENE JORGENSEN

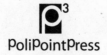

PoliPointPress

14   13   12   11   10   2   3   4   5

Production management: BookMatters, Berkeley
Book design: BookMatters, Berkeley
Cover design: Naylor Design

Library of Congress Cataloging-in-Publication Data has been applied for.

Published by:
PoliPointPress, LLC
80 Liberty Ship Way, Suite 22
Sausalito, CA 94966-3008
(415) 339-4100
www.p3books.com

Distributed by Ingram Publisher Services

Printed in the USA

This book is dedicated to Dean.

Contents

Tables and Figures

Tables

Figures

Boxes

Author's Note

During my illness, I consulted more than a dozen doctors. Some provided exceptional care, for which I am very grateful; others, less so. Several doctors acted unethically, one doctor committed insurance fraud, and another doctor practiced without a medical license. I still rely on some doctors for care; others, I have stopped seeing. I mention no doctors by name, because this book isn't about the specific doctors with whom I came into contact; it is a story about the health care system.

ONE

Paradise Valley

BEWARE OF BEARS! This is the warning that family and friends gave me when they heard I was planning to do some hiking in Montana. They advised me to tie small bells onto my shoes, not to carry any food with me, and never to walk alone; they said I should stay in the car to avoid being mauled by a grizzly bear. Nevertheless, I went to Montana and went hiking, without a companion and without bells. I didn't see a single bear. Instead, I was attacked by something much more menacing than your typical grizzly bear. It was a tiny creature with a ravenous appetite for blood.

I had come to Paradise Valley, in Montana, to attend a conference on the thrilling topic of wolves. Tired after a long day of travel, I decided to take a walk into the hills to get some fresh air and look for wolves. It was an unusually warm April day, with temperatures above 70 degrees, and I soon felt sleepy. I lay down in the fragrant sage bushes for a nap. When I turned my head to the right, I saw a proud bighorn ram on the lookout for female sheep and potential competitors. When I turned my head to the left, I saw a herd of mule deer busily grazing and occasionally raising their heads to survey the surroundings for wolves. The prairie dogs were busy doing what prairie dogs do. I closed my eyes, and before dozing off I thought to myself, "This is Paradise."

Before my trip to Montana, I worked as an economist. When analyzing the wages, pensions, and health benefits of American workers grew tedious, my mind frequently wandered to thoughts of my next hiking trip. I was an active person and enjoyed the outdoors. Nearly every weekend, my husband, my two dogs, and I went hiking in Virginia's mountains. Eventually, I decided to listen to my intuition and went back to school to study a subject that spoke to me: wildlife conservation. The trip to Paradise Valley represented my first step away from being a disgruntled number-crunching economist and toward the establishment of a new and more exciting career. The next day I was scheduled to give a presentation on the costs of government programs that controlled wolf populations below their natural level.

The presentation did not go well. My head was pounding, and I couldn't keep a coherent thought in my mind. I felt feverish and nauseated, and I stumbled around the podium, as if I were drunk. Instead of staying up partying the night before, I had gone to bed early because I had felt exhausted. I slept poorly, nonetheless, twisting and turning in bed. I attributed my malady to nervous anticipation and at the time made no connection to the engorged tick I found behind my left ear at around four o'clock in the morning. Without a second thought, I pulled the tick off, squeezed it between two fingernails, flushed it down the toilet, and went back to bed. My career as a wildlife conservationist ended abruptly that morning in Paradise Valley, before it had even begun.

A New Career

Dermacentor andersoni, more commonly known as the Rocky Mountain wood tick, is less than one-eighth of an inch long, but it possessed the power to change my life forever. Instead of becoming an adventurous conservationist roaming the woods, I became a housebound patient with a mysterious, disabling disease that rendered me unable to work. This book is about my journey through the health care system. It documents my search for a correct diagnosis and proper medical treatment. It also describes my struggle with my health insurance company to ensure it covered my medical expenses. I have been treated by a handful of doctors, including my primary care doctor, an infectious disease doctor, a rheumatologist, a hematologist, and two tick-borne disease specialists. I also consulted a cardiologist, an endocrinologist, and a doctor who specializes in alternative medicine. I have lost gallons of blood to testing and swallowed medication by the bucketful. I have been poked and prodded, and have undergone two minor surgeries. Some doctors spent less than five minutes with me and chalked my illness up to depression or a long-lasting flu, without so much as a passing thought for what I had to say. Other doctors placed nebulous labels on my ailment, such as "chronic fatigue syndrome," or "lupus-like autoimmune disease." Although these doctors validated the fact that I was ill, they simultaneously took away my hope for recovery. Fortunately, the best doctors listened and continued to search for answers until I showed signs of improvement.

Finding good doctors is only half the battle. Paying for their services is the other half. Health care is expensive, even for people with first-rate insurance coverage. My health insurance coverage looks good on paper. My health plan, obtained through my husband's workplace, is with a preferred provider organization (PPO). I have no deductibles, and the copayments are low for in-network services. Moreover, my health plan does not require a referral to see a specialist, nor do I need to get preapproval to see one. If I go outside the plan, it covers 80 percent of out-of-network services . . .

up to a limit. The plan reimburses out-of-network services at a rate that it determines to be "reasonable and customary" in my geographic area. However, the reasonable and customary rate often turned out to be much lower than what my out-of-network physicians customarily charged. As a result, I had to pay 100 percent of the difference.

My prescription coverage has the appearance of being comprehensive but, in fact, leaves much to be desired. The copayments range from $5 to $25 for prescriptions, which I can fill at the pharmacy of my choice. In reality, I end up paying substantially more for prescriptions. My plan has quantity limits on many drugs and does not cover some medications at all. Some drugs, like the sleep medication I was prescribed, have bizarre limitations on coverage. My health plan covers only two out of every three months' supply, so I was left to foot the bill for sleeping pills every third month—or spend a month with little sleep. In the case of certain antibiotics, the plan covers only 10 days of every month, which left me with a choice: I could experience long breaks in treatment with the risk of nurturing a treatment-resistant infection, or pay hundreds of dollars out of pocket.

So, despite my "good" health insurance coverage, my illness ended up costing me a total of $11,058 in medical expenses. More accurately, I paid $11,058, *in addition* to the $7,500 that I paid each year in insurance premiums.

Before I got sick, my health plan covered all claims. After I got sick and started running up health expenses, the health insurance company began turning down claims on a regular basis. Some claims were turned down due to "missing diagnostic codes," or "incomplete doctor tax identification numbers." In other cases, my insurance company sent me on frustrating wild goose chases. I would, for example, receive a request for a copy of the doctor's license. When the doctor refused to comply with my request, I had to contact the state board of medicine to obtain a copy. In other instances, the reason my claim was rejected was unclear.

My mysterious illness rendered me too sick to work. Even everyday tasks, such as shopping and cooking, became too exhausting for me. At times, my illness made me a prisoner in my own bed. But my health insurance company made sure that I was never idle. The mounting health care bills forced me to take up an involuntary, unpaid, part-time job: dealing with the insurance. It involved a tremendous amount of paperwork. Claims had to be filled out, copied, and mailed to the insurance company. A surprisingly large number of claims were never received, or were "lost in the system" and had to be resubmitted. I placed many a phone call to customer service to try to figure out why claims were denied. The "explanation codes" on the statements of benefits were anything but explanatory. Claims that were denied had to be refiled with additional information. The insurance company began demanding pre-authorization for certain drugs, and I had to beg my doctor's office to fill out the necessary paperwork. Sometimes doctors refused to cater to my insurance company's demands.

Following up on insurance matters while I was in good health would have been a daunting task. While I was sick, it was overwhelming. Health insurance companies know that sick people are poorly positioned to deal with complicated and time-consuming insurance matters, and they use this fact to their benefit. Insurance companies regularly turn down insurance claims for no reason, in the hope that patients can't or won't follow up on rejected claims, thus leaving the insurance company off the hook. Because sick patients have the highest expenses, this strategy translates into significant costs savings for insurance companies.

As I look at the small mountain of paperwork made up of invoices from doctors and laboratories, pharmacy receipts, and the ironically named "explanation of benefits," the only comfort I can take is that it could have been worse. A lot worse. If I had not had health insurance coverage, my tests, medical services, and prescription drugs would have cost a whopping $180,000, instead of the $11,058 I paid out of pocket. If I had not had health insurance, my husband and I would have been forced to mortgage our home, drain our retirement savings, and run up credit-card debt, which we would have had no hope of ever repaying.

Paying for health care is a big problem for many American families. One in five of the families surveyed by the Center for Health System Change reported problems paying medical bills.[1] The majority—60 percent—had health insurance but nonetheless accrued substantial debt that often amounted to thousands of dollars.[2] In 2007, about 2.2 million Americans filed for bankruptcy due to medical debt. Moreover, the unaffordability of health care not only affects the pocketbook but adversely affects people's health. According to a Kaiser Family Foundation survey, roughly one in four people—27 percent—said that they or a family member had postponed getting needed health care.[3] About one in five people surveyed—21 percent—said they or a family member did not fill a prescription; and one in seven cut pills, skipped doses of medicine, or both.

The Health Care Mystery

Before my journey through the health care system began, I studied health care as a part of my job as an economist. My knowledge was primarily academic and came largely in the form of statistics and figures. What I did not know, as an economist, but would soon find out as a patient, was how the health care system works for patients. As an economist, I knew that Americans spend over $2.5 trillion a year on health care; as a patient, I discovered just how devastatingly expensive health care can be for the sick.[4] Americans spend $8,160 per person a year on health care expenses, but this is an average. Most people have relatively few expenses in a year, whereas the sick, like me, run up huge expenses.

After my tick bite, the first prescription I filled was for 10 days of antibiotics at a cost of $12.55. But my tick bite turned out to be substantially more expensive, and the duration of treatment was measured in years rather than days. Six years to be exact. Six years of exhaustion and pain. Six years of life stolen. At first, I assumed that the problem would take care of itself; when it did not, I sought medical treatment. It took about a month before I began to suspect that my doctor did not know what was wrong with me and that a cure might be more elusive than I had been led to believe. Another six months passed before I found an experienced physician and got the correct diagnosis. After five years of treatment, my expenses had accumulated to $96,000.

The nation's health care costs are also rising quickly. Since 2001, health care expenditures have increased by 71 percent per person; over the same period, the overall price level, or inflation, increased by 20 percent.[5] This rate of increase is projected to continue so that by 2018, health care expenses will represent 20 percent of the U.S. gross domestic product (GDP). This means that for every dollar, 20 cents will go toward health care. In comparison, Americans spend 10 cents of every dollar on food.[6]

The reasons for the rise in health care costs are complex. As the population ages, the demand for health care rises. Spending on prescription medications is growing as new and more expensive drugs enter the market. Likewise, new medical technologies are being developed that are more effective but also more expensive. For instance, an MRI of the knee costs about 15 times more than an X-ray. [7] However, it also provides more information about the knee, allowing for a more accurate diagnosis.

An aging population and advancements in medical technology do not explain why U.S. health care is so expensive. European countries and Canada also have aging populations and have also adopted the latest scanning technology. Their doctors perform cutting-edge surgeries and prescribe new drugs, just like U.S. doctors. Nonetheless, health care in Europe and Canada costs about half of what it costs in the United States. In 2007, health expenditures averaged $7,290 per person in the United States; Canadians paid $3,895 on average. [8] Norwegians spend more than any other Europeans for their health care: $4,763 per person in 2007; the Brits, in the same year, spent only $2,992 per person. Although these countries spend less, they offer universal coverage. By contrast, in 2009, about 46 million Americans were without any health insurance coverage, according to data from the U.S. Census Bureau. [9] An additional 25 million Americans were underinsured, meaning their insurance did not provide sufficient financial protection against illness. [10]

This book tries to answer the question of why health care is so much more expensive in the United States than in other wealthy countries. As I documented the rapidly accumulating costs of my medical care from the first $12.55 prescription to the total of almost $100,000, I began to notice the waste in resources, the excessive pricing, and the underlying high administrative costs. When I went outside my plan's network to seek care from specialists, the price of a consultation increased two to three times, as out-of-network doctors typically charge substantially higher prices than in-network doctors. Some doctors mistrusted diagnostic tests ordered by previous doctors and repeated the tests with their own preferred laboratory. Other doctors, with preconceived opinions about the underlying cause of my illness, ordered tests they hoped would support their diagnoses. My gynecologist was convinced I had syphilis, despite the fact that I have been happily married for years and that my husband is in perfect health. Every time I saw him, he ordered a syphilis test. Finally, I found a new gynecologist.

The services I received were expensive, but my health plan and I were also repeatedly billed for services that I had never received. Some in-network doctors charged for an extended consultation lasting 40 minutes, even though they had spent less than 15 minutes with me. Laboratories regularly double-billed for tests. The hospital billed for services they never provided me. The unwarranted billing ended up costing my health plan thousands of dollars in extra costs. But these costs are merely a symptom of the underlying problem.

The Book

I started writing this book in the spring of 2006, three years into my treatment. At the time, I was too sick to do much of anything and was confined to my home most of the time. My vision was blurred—my eyes repeatedly focused in and out, like a broken pair of binoculars, making it difficult to read a book or text on the computer screen. I had become extremely light-sensitive and had to wear sunglasses, even on overcast days, when watching TV, or when sitting in front of the computer. I had developed chronic inflammation in my muscles, which felt like a sunburn deep under the skin. Joint pain made holding a pen or typing for more than a few minutes difficult. But the most devastating symptom I had developed was neurological. I felt like a thick fog had settled over my brain, interfering with my ability to think clearly. I had become so forgetful that while I was talking, I would find myself unable to complete the sentence. Writing was even more challenging. I found it hard to formulate what I wanted to say in my head and to translate it into words to be committed to paper or the computer screen. I couldn't retrieve words, and the spelling of common words suddenly seemed unfamiliar. One day I mulled over the spelling of "business" for half an hour; another day it was "research."

Writing a whole book may seem a rather ambitious project for someone who cannot even write a complete sentence. I set out to write just one paragraph a day. In the beginning, I would write about my everyday observations or whatever came to my mind when I sat down in front of my computer. Some days, I was too sick to write at all; other days, I gave up in frustration after writing only a couple of words. Six months into the project, I outlined the first chapter and began to write from the beginning. When I wasn't writing, I was conducting research on health care. Slowly, one paragraph a day, the pages began to fill, and after three years I had a complete book.

This book is based on my personal experiences and shaped by the specifics of my illness, the doctors I sought medical care from, the coverage of my health plan, and ultimately how I saw the world around me through the prism of pain and confusion my illness caused. Still, my experiences will be familiar to anyone who has been unfortunate enough to suffer from a serious medical condition. My hope is that this book will help readers better understand the health care system and help them seek better care for themselves and their families as they navigate their way through the network of health care providers and insurers.

TWO

Health Insurance Industry

DIAGNOSIS

I DON'T REMEMBER MUCH about the rest of my trip to Montana, other than that I spent most of the time in bed. Somehow I managed to drive myself the 100 miles to the airport, check in, get on a plane, change planes in Chicago, and grab a cab to take me home. A couple of days later, I was feeling better, despite swollen lymph nodes that had appeared down my neck like a string of pearls. At my husband's insistence, I reluctantly scheduled an appointment with my doctor. It took less than 10 seconds for him to diagnose me with Lyme disease. He prescribed me a 10-day course of antibiotics.

My doctor further instructed me to contact the Montana Department of Health to inquire about tick-borne diseases present in the state. The Health Department employee I talked to was encouraging. He told me that there was no Lyme disease in Montana and that I had probably come down with the Colorado tick fever and would recover in a matter of days. After having written off Lyme disease as the cause of my illness, I was surprised when the blood test came back positive. I called the Montana Health Department back to inform them that Lyme disease had arrived in their state. This time, the person I spoke to admitted that a handful of people had developed Lyme-like bull's-eye rashes after being bitten by ticks in Paradise Valley. But he insisted that Lyme disease did not exist in Montana. Montana was at the time the only state in the country without a single reported case of Lyme disease, despite occurrences of the disease having been documented in all the bordering states of Wyoming, Idaho, and the Dakotas, as well as in Alberta, Canada.[1]

I had first heard about Lyme disease 10 years earlier from a tropical disease specialist in New York City, whom I had consulted after becoming sick during a trip to the Central American country of Belize. When I told him that I had an upcoming conference to attend in Connecticut, he strongly warned me against going. He told me about a terrifying bacterial infection in that state, which, he said, destroys the nervous system, disabling people so severely they cannot get out of bed. The disease eventually results in death if left untreated. And the most incredible part was that it is caused by a bite from a tick. I found it hard to believe that a disease worse than most tropical diseases, and one I had never heard of, should exist in a tranquil place like Connecticut. So I ignored the doctor's warning and went to Connecticut, though I did adhere to his advice of staying out of tall grass and scrub, walking in the middle of the path, and checking myself for ticks. One year later I read an article in the *New York Times* about Lyme disease and realized that the tropical disease specialist was not crazy, just better informed than most doctors.[2]

By the end of the 10-day antibiotic treatment I had not recovered. In fact, I was feeling worse and had developed new, troublesome symptoms: I had numbness in my legs and feet, throbbing sensations in my muscles, loss of muscle control in my face, and sensations of pressure in spots on the top of my head as if someone were pressing a finger hard against my scalp. My brain functions had further deteriorated, and I couldn't formulate a coherent thought. My primary care doctor referred me to an infectious disease specialist at a prestigious university research hospital in Washington DC. The specialist diagnosed me with chronic neurological Lyme disease and recommended three weeks of intravenous (IV) antibiotic therapy. He also tested me for a couple of other tick-borne infections, but the tests came back negative.

Soon after I received the diagnosis of chronic neurological Lyme disease, my insurance woes began. My health insurance company refused to cover the cost of the insertion of the IV tube to administer the medication. The doctor was on the phone shouting for a good 20 minutes while I pondered the waste of this highly paid infectious disease specialist's time. The insurance company did not budge and insisted that the IV tube be inserted by its home nursing company.

The home nursing company insisted that I travel to its facility in the far suburbs. I explained that my neurological illness had rendered me too sick to drive a car. In fact, I could barely get out of bed. Three days later, and after numerous calls to the home nursing company, to my health plan, and to the doctor, the home nursing company agreed to send a nurse to my home. This delay in treatment was caused solely by the insurance company's attempt to steer me into the lowest-cost treatment option rather than the one based on medical considerations. Although the research hospital is an in-network hospital, its rates were substantially higher than those my health plan had negotiated with the home nursing company.

Restrictions on Care

Restrictions on coverage of medical services are not uncommon. Insurance plans routinely require referrals to see specialists and pre-authorization for certain medical services, deny coverage for treatments deemed experimental, and refuse to cover a long list of medical procedures. Prescription-drug coverage has restrictions on dosage and quantity per prescription and sets limits on the duration of treatment. These sorts of limitations can make it difficult for patients to obtain the needed medical care ordered by their physicians.

Health insurance is supposed to protect against costs associated with medical problems. An insurance company spreads the risk across a large number of people to offset the high cost of covering sick people by the gains from insuring healthy people who incur few expenses. Some health insurance plans cover only catastrophic health events, leaving the insurance holder to pay for normal medical expenses, such as doctor consultations and prescription medications. More commonly, health insurance plans cover a wide range of medical-related expenses.

But health insurance is more than just insurance. It also gives insurance holders access to lower prices. Insurance companies, representing thousands of patients, have the clout to bargain for favorable prices with health care providers in their network. Individuals without insurance end up paying full prices for the same services. The requested price may be quite different from the negotiated price. For example, the negotiated price for a cardiologist I consulted in 2006 was nearly half of the standard charge, and the negotiated prices for tests with the two diagnostic laboratories in my plan's network were only a seventh of the price they charged patients without insurance.

Two problems are inherent in any type of insurance, whether it be fire, flood, or health insurance: moral hazard and adverse selection. Moral hazard arises when the insured parties (in this case, patients) do not bear the full consequences of their actions.

In the case of auto insurance, people may drive less carefully when they are not financially liable for accidents. In the case of health insurance, a person may engage in more risky behavior if the resulting health care is covered by insurance. Health insurance companies deal with moral hazard by having subscribers pay a share of the costs through copayments and deductibles.

Adverse selection results when healthy people opt out of purchasing insurance while sick people opt in. The result is that insured people tend to be sicker and incur higher costs than the general population. Insurance companies protect themselves against adverse selection by denying coverage to people with pre-existing conditions and dumping people from their plans who develop serious medical problems. The result is that people who need health insurance the most are often not eligible in the private market. In 2006, Blue Shield of California came under investigation for rescinding coverage due to minor omissions on applications.[3] Essentially, Blue Shield enrolled people and collected premium payments only to cancel the policies after the policy holders got sick. Dropped by their plans, these people—who badly needed coverage—were either unable to purchase insurance or faced exorbitant premiums.

Another example of how the health insurance system fails its customers can be found in a story featured in the *New York Times* about Vicki Readling, a real estate agent who, despite an annual income of $60,000, could not afford health insurance.[4] Like most real estate agents, Ms. Readling worked as an independent contractor and therefore did not have access to employer-provided health insurance. In 2005, Ms. Readling was diagnosed with breast cancer and underwent successful treatment. When her health insurance policy expired at the end of the year, she was not able to renew the policy. The combination of expensive cancer-prevention medications and the risk of a relapse of cancer classified her as a high-cost person. She applied for health insurance with other companies, but they refused to offer her insurance. The one insurance company that was willing to insure her charged $2,300 per month in premiums for an insurance plan with a deductible of $5,000. That meant that she would have had to pay $32,600 a year before receiving a single dollar in benefits.

Recognizing the failure of the market to provide health coverage to the elderly and the disabled—who tend to be more sick and have higher health care expenses—Congress established the Medicare program in 1965. Its sister program, Medicaid, provides health coverage for low-income people. Medicare is a public health insurance program. Funded by payroll taxes of current workers, it pays for medical services for people who are 65 and older, as well as disabled individuals. Medicare has been hugely successful in providing health coverage for the elderly. Less than 2 percent of people 65 and older have no health coverage, whereas in 2008, 20.3 percent of Americans aged 18 to 64 were without coverage.[5]

While Medicare, Medicaid, and SCHIP (State Children's Health Insurance Program) have been fairly successful in covering the populations they serve, private health insurance companies have become increasingly unsuccessful. The market-based approach to health insurance is failing one in every four Americans. A total of 46 million Americans are without any health insurance coverage.[6] An additional 35 million go without health insurance for part of the year.[7] Not only have private health insurance companies failed to reach out to uninsured people, but they have dropped, on net, 24 million people over the last two decades. In 1988, 74.7 percent of the population had private health coverage; in 2008, only 66.7 percent did. The sharpest drop was in direct-purchase

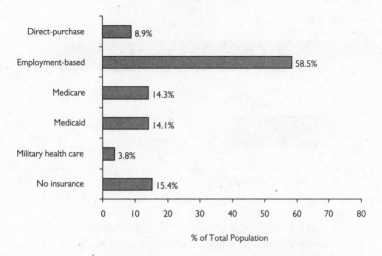

FIGURE 2.1 Health insurance coverage by type of insurance plan: Percentage of total population, 2008.

Source: U.S. Census Bureau 2009: Table C-1. Numbers add up to more than 100% because some people have more than one form of insurance.

insurance, but health coverage through the workplace also declined (see figure 2.1).

Insurance Against Sickness

Employment-based health insurance is the most common type of health insurance in the United States. Nearly 60 percent of Americans have insurance through their workplaces.[8] However, being employed does not guarantee access to employer-provided health insurance. According to the Bureau of Labor Statistics (BLS), three in ten workers worked for employers who did not offer any health insurance.[9] One in four workers who were offered health coverage either could not afford or chose not to participate in their employers' health insurance plans.

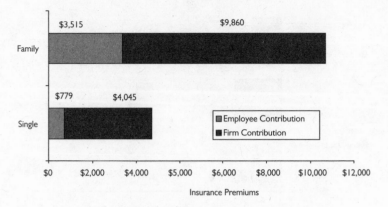

FIGURE 2.2 Average annual firm and employee premium
contributions for single and family coverage, 2009
Source: Kaiser Family Foundation 2009b: Exhibits 6.3, 6.4.

As of 2009, the law does not require employers to offer health
insurance to their employees, and about 40 percent of private companies in the United States do not.[10] Providing health coverage to
employees is expensive. In 2009, the average annual premium for
individual coverage was $4,824, or $400 per month.[11] For family
coverage, premiums were substantially higher, at $13,375 (see fig-
ure 2.2). Most employers pay part of the premium, few employers
pay all of it, and some employers pay nothing. Perversely, high-paid
professional workers are more likely than low-wage service and
sales workers to receive health insurance through their employers,
and they generally pay a smaller share of their insurance premiums. As a result, coverage rates are much higher among high-wage
workers than low-wage workers.[12]

Health insurance can quickly become costly, in particular
for small businesses, when illness strikes. A bookstore in Kansas
had its health insurance premium raised by 28 percent for *all* 36
employees after *one* employee became sick with emphysema.[13] Even

after the death of the employee, the insurance premiums continued to increase for several years. The bookstore changed insurance carriers, only to face additional increases in premiums after another employee became sick with stomach cancer. Essentially, the bookstore was punished financially for choosing to retain seriously ill employees rather than firing them in their time of greatest need.

During the first decade of the 21st century, the annual premiums for employer-provided health coverage have more than doubled, and providing health coverage to employees is an increasingly large burden for businesses. The $4,824 annual premium for single coverage in 2009 was 120 percent higher than the $2,196 price in 1999. [14] In comparison, inflation increased by 29 percent and median nominal wages by 35 percent over the same period.[15] Due to the rising cost of premiums, many employers have been forced to cut back on coverage, drop family coverage, or stop offering coverage altogether if they want to stay in business.

Managed Care

In the "good old days" of health care in the 1960s, most people with health insurance had indemnity insurance. Indemnity insurance is a fee-for-service insurance that reimburses health care providers for medical services. The traditional plans had no built-in cost containment measures, and health care expenditures were increasing rapidly. Congress's solution to rising health care costs was to pass the Health Maintenance Organization (HMO) Act of 1973, which required companies with 25 or more employees that already offered health insurance, to also offer an HMO plan. HMOs were initially set up as not-for-profit organizations that emphasized preventive care, such as vaccinations, disease screening, and disease-prevention education. Preventive care was supposed to translate into better health and a diminished demand for medical care.

The HMO Act of 1973 successfully established managed care, but was less successful at curtailing the rise in health care costs. In 1973, national health expenditures accounted for 7.2 percent of gross domestic product (GDP).[16] In the following decades, health care costs continued to grow much faster than the economy. By 2008, national health expenditures accounted for more than 16 percent of GDP. The federal Centers for Medicare and Medicaid Services (CMS) projects that by 2018, 20 percent of our economic activity in this country will be related to health care.

In 1973, "health maintenance" sounded like a good idea. But managing patients' care turned out to be terribly expensive. HMOs employ their own full staff of physicians and nurses to review and make critical decisions regarding patient care. The staff authorizes referrals to specialists and for nonstandard tests, pre-certify nonemergency hospital admission and outpatient surgery, and make determinations about whether a certain drug or procedure is "medically necessary." They never see the patients but regularly overrule the recommendations of the patients' own doctors.[17] About 50 percent of appeals for medical treatment that were initially denied by HMO plans in Texas were overturned by the appeals board. This suggests that insurance companies routinely deny patients medical treatment that is medically necessary.

Managing health care is bureaucratic and requires huge amounts of paperwork to be shuffled around to monitor the use of medical resources by physicians and patients. For example, requests are denied, patients appeal the decisions, physicians send additional information to the HMO, and cases are reconsidered by a review committee. The administrative costs of private for-profit health insurance companies are estimated at 10 to 25 percent, which is much higher than administrative costs for nonprofit and public plans, such as Medicare.[18]

Another reason managed care ultimately failed to rein in health care expenditures is that most HMOs operate as profit-maximizing companies rather than the nonprofit organizations envisioned by Congress in 1973. UnitedHealth Group, Aetna Inc., and WellPoint Inc. are for-profit corporations whose stocks are publicly traded on the stock exchange. Their CEOs are paid generous compensation packages just like CEOs at other large American corporations. According to *Forbes* magazine, the United-Health's CEO, William W. McGuire, was the third-highest paid CEO in America in 2005; he had a total compensation of $125 million—most of it in stock options.[19]

Finally, the intent of the HMO Act of 1973 was to make preventive care one of the core principles of HMOs. Within the profit-maximizing paradigm of managed care, however, preventive care is seen as a bad investment. Due to the transitory nature of the insurance market, where patients regularly change jobs and insurance carriers, insurance companies have short time horizons. As a result, few HMOs are willing to invest in preventive care because they are unlikely to reap the benefits.

In the mid-nineties, HMOs were the most common type of private health plan. But their restrictive structure—requiring members to stay within the network, assigning primary care physicians as gatekeepers, and micromanaging patients' care—made them increasingly unpopular. By 1999, PPOs overtook HMOs as the preferred type of employer-provided coverage. PPO plans offer patients more choices and do not cost much more than HMOs. In

BOX 1

Common Types of Health Insurance Plans

HMO: Health Maintenance Organization plans require a patient to choose a primary care physician who is in charge of the patient's care. People with HMO plans have to get referrals from primary care physicians to see specialists or for non-emergency procedures. HMO plans cover only in-network services and rarely reimburse for outside network services.

PPO: Preferred Provider Organization plans are less restrictive than HMOs and typically cover a larger network of physicians and facilities. Some PPOs require referrals for specialists and some elective procedures, but many plans allow for self-referral. Patients with a PPO can go outside the network for services, but they will pay a higher copay, typically a percentage of the service rate.

POS: Point of Service plans fall between HMOs and PPOs. Like HMO plans, POS plans have primary care physicians acting as gatekeepers for other medical services; however, POS plans allow patients to go outside the network. The copayment for out-of-network services is typically much higher for POS plans than PPO plans.

EPO: Exclusive Provider Organization plans are a type of man-aged care plan similar to HMO plans. People with an EPO plan have a primary care physician and need referrals to other health services. EPOs typically have a small network of doctors and do not cover out-of-network services. EPOs focus on preventive care and encourage people to take steps to stay healthy. The biggest difference between EPOs and HMOs is their contractual arrangements with health care providers. EPOs pay physicians based on services provided, whereas HMOs pay a fixed monthly fee based on patient base.

SDHP: Self-Directed Health Plans are similar to PPOs but typically have high deductibles for nonroutine care. Self-directed plans have the added feature of a self-directed account (SDA). The plan "deposits" a quarterly allowance into the account—around $250 per quarter—to be used for routine and preventive health care services. As long as a person stays within the quarterly allowance, he or she does not incur any extra expenses for health care services covered by the account. Unused funds in the account can be rolled over to the next quarter. SDHPs are typically cheaper than PPOs, but have higher deductibles.

HDHP with Health Savings Accounts: High-Deductible Health Plans are a more affordable (or less unaffordable) type of health insurance. As the name implies, the plans have high deductibles of at least $1,150 for single coverage and $2,300 for family coverage. HDHPs have lower premiums than other types of health plans and are an attractive option for young and healthy people with typically few health expenses who wish to insure against serious health events.

HSA: Health Savings Accounts give people the option to save tax-free to pay for future health expenses. People with an HSA can deposit a certain amount of pretax earnings into the savings account to pay for health care. Money not used is rolled over to the next year and earns tax-free interest.

2009, the average annual premium for employer-provided HMO individual plans was $4,878, compared to $4,922 for PPO plans.[20]

The Explanation of Benefits

In the middle of my IV antibiotic treatment, I received a bill for $660 from the laboratory that had done the blood tests for Lyme and other tick-borne diseases. My first response was to cry. After wiping the tears away—I felt overwhelmed by my illness, and now this—I felt outrage. The lab fee is covered under my insurance plan and, theoretically, I should only pay a $10 copayment. When I called the laboratory's billing department, I was first told that I did not have health insurance. When I insisted that I did, I was told that my insurance did not cover tests from this laboratory and that I should pay the bill in full and seek reimbursement from my health plan. Finally, I talked to a supervisor who agreed to submit the claim to my insurance.

When I received the explanation of benefits statement from my insurance company, I understood why the laboratory was so eager to bill me directly instead of my insurance company. It turns out that my health insurance company had negotiated prices with the laboratory that are substantially lower than the prices I was being charged. My health plan paid only $69 for the tests for which I had been billed $660. The laboratory stood to earn almost 10 times more by billing me rather than the insurance company.

At first glance, the explanation of benefits statements are nearly incomprehensible. They include long lists of dollar amounts, six columns with different—seemingly unrelated—figures, followed by incomprehensible three-digit explanation codes. For example, code "233" explains that "this claim has been paid in conjunction with the authorization on file," while code "889" notes that "per diems left in auth(5) cannot cover this claim-per-diem," followed by a code "MPR" for "multi-plan return queue." This mumbo jumbo activated my economic mind, and I began tracking my medical expenses in a spreadsheet to determine the costs of my illness.

Once I learned to decipher the codes, the explanation of benefits statements became a trove of information. The "requested charge" is the amount that physicians, hospitals, and laboratories charge for the medical services provided. The "allowable charge" is, in the case of in-network providers, the agreed-upon fee set by the insurance company. In the case of out-of-network providers, the allowable charge is the "reasonable and customary rate" as determined by the insurance company itself.

The reasonable and customary rate is what the health plan determines to be the going fee for a doctor consultation or medical procedure in a geographic area. However, they were often set unreasonably low, way below what doctors customarily charge in my area, leaving me responsible for the difference. For example, if my doctor charges me $300 for a consultation, and my plan determines that the reasonable and customary rate is $200, I pay $100 plus my $40 copay (20 percent of $200).

In 2007, the New York attorney general opened an investigation into whether my insurance company and four other companies were setting their reasonable and customary rates too low. Each of the companies under investigation used data provided by the health care research company Ingenix, which is a subsidiary of UnitedHealth Group, the largest insurance company in the country and one of the five being investigated. The attorney general's investigation revealed that insurers use distorted data from Ingenix to lowball local market rates for various types of physician services and thereby keep reimbursement costs down.

The attorney general estimated that Ingenix underestimates rates by as much as 28 percent.[21]

In early 2009, UnitedHealth settled with New York's attorney general. The company did not admit to any wrongdoing but agreed to overhaul its databases and pay $350 million to settle a class-action suit.[22] A new database to calculate reasonable and customary rates, funded by UnitedHealth, will be set up and run by an independent university.

As my medical expenses accumulated and the pile of bills, invoices, and explanation of benefits statements grew, the columns of numbers in my spreadsheet got longer. The first prescription of 10 days of antibiotics cost $12.55. The bills for three weeks of IV treatment came to a staggering $4,500. Before the year was over, my medical expenses were almost $7,500. Five years after the tick bite, my insurance company and I had paid out a total of $96,000.

Despite good-on-paper insurance coverage, I got stuck paying substantially more than my copays for the health care I received. After five years, my out-of-pocket costs had accumulated to $11,058. My only consolation is that without insurance, the same care would have cost me about $180,000.[23]

Insurance Failures

The birthplace of managed care is the Coulee Dam in Washington state. At the time of its completion in 1939, the Coulee Dam was considered the Eighth Wonder of the World and to this day, remains the largest concrete structure in the United States. Industrialist Henry J. Kaiser, who made his money in concrete, was put in charge of building the dam. In the early 1930s, Mr. Kaiser met a doctor named Sidney Garfield, who operated a small 12-bed hospital in the Mojave Desert, which provided hospital care and preventive care on a prepaid basis. Mr. Kaiser was impressed with Dr. Garfield's managed care and invited him to set up a similar program for the 6,500 workers building the Coulee Dam. Mr. Kaiser paid Dr. Garfield a fixed amount per worker to treat accident cases, and workers contributed an additional 20 cents out of their monthly wages for other medical services.[24] Mr. Kaiser expanded health care coverage to the workers in his shipyards during World War II. After the war ended, he opened up his health plan to the public and established Kaiser Permanente. Today 8.6 million people have health coverage with Kaiser Permanente.[25]

During the war, other employers followed suit. The federal government had imposed wage and price controls to rein in the inflation resulting from a shortage of both consumer goods and workers.[26] Millions of workers were joining the military, and employers were having difficulty attracting enough workers. A nonwage benefit, such as health insurance, was considered noninflationary and did not violate the wage control law. The foundation was laid for the system that we have today of employer-provided health care through private health insurance. More a fluke of history than a well-thought-out system, this model is not a particularly effective way to provide health care as only employed people and their families can obtain health coverage. People who become seriously ill and lose their jobs often also lose their health coverage at the time when they need it the most. [27]

In our employment-based health insurance system, people without jobs are not the only ones left without coverage. About 30 percent of workers do not have coverage through their employers, either because their employers do not offer coverage or because the workers do not qualify, which is the case for many part-time and temporary workers.[28] Private health insurance companies do offer health insurance for direct purchase, but many people either do

BOX 2

How to Appeal a Denied Claim with a Health Insurance Company

1 When you receive a letter or "explanation of benefits" statement rejecting a claim, call your insurance agency immediately to find out why. Sometimes, claim requests are turned down for easily correctable mistakes, such as a missing diagnosis code. Most insurance plans make patients responsible for getting the missing information and correcting any mistakes. During this phone call, you should try to obtain three pieces of information: a) why the claim was rejected; b) which information you need to obtain (ask for specifics); and c) how to request an appeal. If the service representative does not answer your questions to your satisfaction, ask to speak to a supervisor.

Don't delay making contact. Insurance plans have strict timelines, and failure to meet these usually makes you responsible for the bill by default.

2 If you receive a bill from a physician or laboratory that you think is incorrect, call the billing department to find out why you are being billed. If the physician or laboratory is in-network, it cannot bill you for more than your copayment (after the deductible), even if your insurance plan refuses to pay for the service provided. In the case of out-of-network providers, you may be without recourse; you are responsible for the full amount if your plan does not cover a service.

3. If pre-authorization is denied, call and find out why the pre-authorization was not granted. If the requested service is not considered "medically necessary," you will need to ask your doctor for a second request and additional supporting information, such as test results or observations of your condition deteriorating. Sometimes a second opinion helps.

4. The next step is to write a formal letter of appeal. Address the letter to the medical director. (Call to find out who it is.) Jason Theodosakis and David T. Feinberg, in their book *Don't Let Your HMO Kill You*, provide a nice sample letter requesting an appeal that can easily be modified to fit any situation.

5. If your appeal is denied, appeal again until you have exhausted the appeal process. Also, talk to your physician about alternative treatments. If the alternatives are unacceptable to you, your last resort is legal action. This can be very time consuming, expensive, and emotionally stressful.

In the case of appealing a denial, persistence often pays off. Insurance companies often reject requests for pre-authorizations and claims but will reconsider if the person is persistent. Unfortunately, appealing a denial can be very difficult for a patient with a serious medical condition. Moreover, to be told that one's medical condition does not warrant the medical procedure that was recommended can be mentally devastating. If you cannot effectively deal with the insurance issues yourself, ask a family member or friend to help you.

not qualify for coverage due to preexisting medical conditions or they cannot afford the premiums. Lack of affordable insurance coverage is without doubt the biggest failure of our private-based health care system.

Underinsurance and lack of insurance lead to undertreatment. We already know from the survey conducted by the Kaiser Family Foundation that 27 percent of the respondents said that they or their family members had postponed getting needed health care because of costs.[29] People treat a wide range of ailments with an aspirin or turn to untested herbal products for relief. In the same survey, 35 percent said that they had relied on home remedies or over-the-counter drugs instead of going to see a doctor.

With the decline in health coverage, medical care increasingly takes place in the emergency room after the medical condition has already spiraled out of control. Uninsured people account for nearly one-fifth of ER visits, and low-income people account for one-third of these visits.[30] In 2009, Providence Hospital in Washington DC reported ER visits increased 13 percent over a single year; feeling the effects of the economic recession, people turned to the ER instead of a primary care physician for care.[31] But many conditions cannot be effectively treated at the ER. Take the case of asthma. Asthma is potentially a very serious medical condition, which can result in brain damage and sometimes death. However, in most cases, the condition can be managed by consulting a physician, minimizing exposure to triggers, and taking medication that reduces inflammation of the airways. But treatment is expensive, prohibitively so for people without insurance. The result is poor management of the condition, as well as a significant increase in the risk of acute asthma attacks and frequent trips to the ER.

From an economic perspective, emergency care—instead of primary and preventive care—results not only in worse health outcomes of the affected populations but also in an inefficient allocation of scarce resources. Long lines in emergency rooms, rationing of services for the uninsured and underinsured, and higher costs of care are some of the immediate consequences. Money that could be spent on other things, such as private consumption, education, and creating new businesses, is instead being sucked up by our inefficient health care system. It is projected that health care expenses will make up a fifth of the total economy by 2018.[32]

The costs to individuals are even greater. Preventive care and primary care translate directly into better health outcomes, higher quality of life, and longer lives. In a study on preventable death among 19 leading industrialized nations, the United States ranked dead last. The researchers estimated that more than 100,000 deaths could be prevented every year if the U.S. health care system performed as well as the French, Japanese, or Australian health care systems.[33] All in all, Americans are getting a pretty bad deal when it comes to health care.

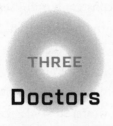

THREE

Doctors

MEDICAL OPINION

"YOU ARE CURED." How I had been longing to hear these sweet little words from my infectious disease doctor. I had completed three weeks of IV antibiotic treatment, and I was feeling much better. Most of my neurological problems had dissolved, my brain was working again, my vision had improved, and the muscle twitching was gone. The doctor warned me that I would probably continue to feel unwell for a while, but it wasn't a cause for concern. Post–Lyme disease syndrome—where patients continue to be sick after the infection has cleared—is a common occurrence in Lyme patients. He told me to return in six months if I wasn't well. When I asked for a follow-up appointment, he refused to schedule one.

In my excitement over being cured, I went out and bought a new pair of running shoes and started planning my next marathon. But I found it was surprisingly hard to return to running. After about half a mile my legs would feel as if they were filled with lead. The fatigue I felt was worse than the fatigue I experienced running an actual marathon. Over the following week, the distance before I needed a rest steadily decreased from one mile to a short run around the block. Some of my other symptoms also returned. I had a constant burning sensation in my muscles, which felt like a sunburn under my skin. My neck was stiff, and bending it was painful. During the night, I would wake up soaked in sweat, despite the cold air the air conditioner was blasting into the bedroom. Ironically, during the day I would be freezing cold, even when wearing a sweater in 90-degree heat with nearly 100 percent humidity.

The list of symptoms continued to grow over the next two months. I developed a chronic sore throat, my right knee became swollen again, and my heart would occasionally skip a beat. Then one day I noticed bright red dots that looked like blood scattered on the bathroom floor. But when I tried to wipe them up, nothing was there to wipe. Relieved there was no blood, I ignored my symptoms, confident in the infectious disease doctor's prediction that I was merely suffering from post–Lyme disease syndrome.

I continued to ignore these symptoms until I came across an article in the *Washington Post* about Amy Tan, one of my favorite authors, and her battle with Lyme disease.[1] Like me, Amy Tan had developed a long list of neurological symptoms, including hallucinations that were even more startling than my blood drops. According to the article, she saw a naked man in her bedroom. She underwent a battery of tests for rare diseases and even had surgery before finally being diagnosed with Lyme disease. The article explained that there is a disagreement over the treatment of Lyme disease in the medical community. Some Lyme disease specialists believe that in the case of chronic infections with neurological manifestations, three weeks of antibiotic therapy is not always sufficient to eradicate the Lyme bacteria from the body. When I read this, I almost choked on my morning coffee. Could it be that my own treatment had failed and I was relapsing?

It certainly made sense. After all, nothing had quite added up when I was diagnosed by the infectious disease specialist. I had become acutely sick after the Montana tick bite, but not a single case of Lyme disease has ever been reported in Montana. I had no bull's-eye rash at the bite site, but I tested positive for Lyme disease.[2] Moreover, the infectious disease doctor had speculated that, based on my blood tests, I was infected several months before my trip to Montana. But how many months? I developed sleeplessness about four months before the Montana trip. After having been a sound sleeper my whole life, I began to lay awake hour after hour every night. Around the same time, my memory started deteriorating. I wrote my loss of memory off to lack off sleep, but I still worried about an early onset of Alzheimer's disease, which had claimed the lives of two grandparents. The previous summer, I had developed muscle twitching in my right thigh. The summer before that I had become light sensitive and had to wear sunglasses outside, even on overcast days.

I was also suffering from recurrent inflammation in my knee. If my knee problems were due to Lyme bacteria feasting on the joint tissue, the infection dated back at least three years. Could it be that my various, seemingly unrelated, medical problems had a common root? But if that were the case, why did I get sick in Montana? I needed answers. The same day I read about Amy Tan, I called the International Lyme and Associated Diseases Society (ILADS), a medical society mentioned in the Tan article, to get a recommendation for a Lyme disease specialist. I was in luck. There was a specialist practicing just a few miles from where I lived. I got an appointment six weeks later.

Outside the Network

I had trusted the infectious disease specialist at the renowned research hospital to provide the best care. But, according to Amy Tan, that trust may have been misplaced. The infectious disease doctor was not a specialist in tick-borne diseases and had limited knowledge of the complexities of this specific class of diseases. Therefore, he had treated me according to narrowly defined treatment guidelines for Lyme disease without considering that my case may not be typical. The doctor had not informed me about alternative treatment protocols and may have been unaware of them. The Tan article convinced me that only a doctor specializing in tick-borne diseases would have sufficient knowledge to get me well again. Luckily, my PPO plan allowed me to go outside the network to seek a second opinion from a physician who had this knowledge.

The Lyme disease specialist did not take any insurance, which allowed him to set his own fees. He spent as much time with his patients as was necessary, and he did not have insurance companies looking over his shoulder. I didn't realize it at the time, but I would soon discover that the network status and the payment structure of health plans significantly affect patient care. In an HMO, physicians are either hired directly or by a medical group that has an exclusive arrangement with the HMO, or they have their own practices that contract with the HMO. Some HMOs allow physicians with their own practices to contract with other HMOs and PPOs, though others have exclusivity agreements. Remuneration in HMO plans is based on a system of capitation (a fixed monthly payment based on the number of patients the physician has). In addition, the physician may also receive performance bonuses, profit sharing, and stock options.

On the other hand, physicians in a PPO group are paid only when patients show up for care. The PPO plan sets predetermined rates that in-network physicians can charge for medical services. These two systems create different incentive structures for physicians. PPO physicians prosper from sick patients who need frequent consultations, while sicker patients create more work for HMO physicians and generate little additional revenue. Patients with chronic illnesses are a steady source of income for PPO physicians, and they are happy to take such patients. The downside of the fee-per-service model is that it creates an incentive to provide excessive services.

HMO and PPO physicians are generally paid less than independent physicians. So, why would they be willing to sign on with managed care plans when as independent physicians they can set their own fees and face no restrictions from insurance companies regarding care? The answer is that HMOs and PPOs give doctors access to a large patient pool. Physicians who contract with HMOs can make up the fee difference in patient volume.[3] As a result, consultation time is reduced and time-consuming tasks, such as taking detailed patient history and physical exams, are replaced by diagnostic testing. Physicians with time constraints will often refer patients to specialists for anything more unusual than the flu. Referral is a quick and easy way for a physician to deal with a sick patient, as it takes less than one minute to write up a referral. In my own experience, out-of-network physicians are less likely to pass patients on to specialists for trivial matters and are more willing to provide the care themselves.

Out-of-network physicians not only cost more money but also require the patient to spend time pursuing claims with the insurance company. In-network physicians are responsible for filing insurance claims and receiving payment from the insurance company and cannot legally charge patients for fees not covered by the insurance. My in-network primary care doctor had a billing department with several full-time employees whose job was to file patient claims with insurance companies, resubmit denied claims, and collect payments from patients with no coverage. Out-of-network doctors essentially subcontract such insurance matters to their patients.

Pursuing insurance claims can be both frustrating and time-consuming. Occasionally, a diagnosis or test code will go missing or be illegible, and the doctor or laboratory must provide the correct information. On several occasions, my insurance plan requested my out-of-network physicians to submit copies of their state medical licenses, certifications, or letters of credentialing/ accreditation, even though I had previously provided them with these copies. Over a six-month period in 2006, my insurance company misplaced more than half the claims I submitted. Beginning in February 2007, reimbursements were regularly delayed. After filing a claim for out-of-network services, I would often receive a letter stating "the health plan needs additional time to review your claim(s) and expects to render a decision within 15 days." Reimbursement usually took considerably longer than the expected 15-day delay.

Blood Parasites

While waiting for the appointment with the Lyme-disease specialist, I began to read up on Lyme disease. What I discovered surprised me. There are two schools of thought about Lyme disease. One argues that Lyme disease is a simple bacterial infection that can easily be treated with a few weeks of antibiotics. The other finds Lyme disease to be extremely complex. The *Borrelia burgdorferi* (*Bb*) bacterium causing Lyme disease is made up of a large number of genes and can take several different forms, including a dormant cyst form that allows the bug to hide from the body's immune system.[4] According to this school of thought, extended treatment is required to cure a chronic infection. Experts cannot even agree upon what constitutes a cure. Many patients with Lyme disease continue to have symptoms after the completion of therapy. Proponents of short-term therapy argue that these symptoms are due to what they call post–Lyme disease syndrome, not an active infection. Others argue that persistent and returning symptoms result from an active infection and that continued antibiotic therapy can therefore be helpful.

I further learned that the Lyme spirochetes can interfere with the immune system, making an infected person susceptible to other tick-borne infections.[5] The black-legged ticks that transmit Lyme disease are also a vector for other diseases with exotic names, such as babesiosis, anaplasmosis, and bartonellosis.[6] Therefore, people infected with Lyme disease are often coinfected with another tick-borne disease as well.[7] In Paradise Valley, Montana, where I was bitten, a mysterious tick-borne disease had recently been discovered. It was a "Lyme-like" infection in which people developed a bull's-eye rash but never tested positive for Lyme disease.[8] Health officials did not know what caused the infection or how to treat it.

By the time my appointment with the Lyme-disease specialist finally came around, I had read up on tick-borne infections, and I arrived with a long list of questions. The doctor spent more than half an hour going over my symptom history, another half hour doing a physician exam, and to my delight took the time to answer my questions. The Lyme disease specialist concurred with the infectious disease doctor that I did have chronic neurological

Lyme disease but disagreed that it had been cured with three
weeks of antibiotics. Based on the fact that symptoms had reap-
peared after completion of treatment, he was certain that I had
relapsed. His diagnosis was confirmed by a highly positive Lyme
test.

He also tested me for about a dozen other tick-borne diseases.
The test for a rare West Coast strain of *Babesia*, only known as
WA-1, came back highly positive.[9] Babesiosis is caused by a blood
parasite called piroplasms. The *Babesia* piroplasms hide within
red blood cells, and the liver is a favorite organ to colonize. Over
time, the piroplasms can invade every organ of the body, including the heart. When the heart becomes infected, congestive heart
failure and death can result. The mortality rate of babesiosis is 10
percent in the United States and 50 percent in Europe among
symptomatic patients.[10]

Babesiosis was first discovered in 1888 by its namesake, Dr.
Victor Babes, who studied cattle diseases in Romania. More than
100 strains of *Babesia* have been identified around the world.[11]
The first reported case of babesiosis (*B. divergens*) in humans was
a Yugoslavian farmer in 1957. A different strain, *B. microti*, sur-
faced in Nantucket in 1969 and was named Nantucket Fever. The
name was subsequently dropped after lobbying from the island's
residents, who did not want to have their quaint island associated with a deadly disease. By the 1980s, human babesiosis was
reported up and down the East Coast. Then, in 1991, my novel
West Coast strain (now named *B. duncani*) was discovered in
the state of Washington. Soon, cases showed up in Oregon and
California as well.[12]

My diagnosis of babesiosis both relieved and upset me. I was
relieved to know that I had finally gotten a diagnosis on the illness
that I had contracted from the tick bite in Montana. The diagnosis

also explained why my initial intravenous antibiotic treatment had failed so miserably. Babesiosis is not a bacterial infection like Lyme disease, and therefore antibiotics will generally be ineffective.[13] But I was also very upset. I had been sick for nine long months before finally beginning treatment.

Patients as Consumers

My experiences changed me from a passive patient, who expected the physician to have all the answers and rarely make mistakes, to an active patient, who stayed informed about my medical conditions by reading books and journal articles. Anyone with a computer has easy access to medical abstracts for free through the National Institutes of Health (NIH) (www.PubMed.gov). Before the Internet, access to medical information was restricted to libraries connected to medical schools and medical journals with expensive subscriptions. Nowadays, with a few mouse clicks, anybody can download medical journal articles for a fee, typically ranging from $10 to $30. Medical societies and patient advocacy groups also produce educational materials for the general public, which can be found by conducting a simple Google search.

Moreover, drug companies are actively encouraging people to become active consumers. Television viewers are bombarded with ads that encourage them to ask their doctors about drug X. Through advertisements, drug companies make people aware of new medical conditions and encourage patients to use their drugs to treat common ailments. A survey by Harvard School of Public Health, Kaiser Family Foundation, and *USA TODAY* found that 32 percent of Americans have asked their doctors about a particular drug after seeing it advertised.[14] According to those surveyed, physicians wrote prescriptions for 44 percent of the cases where the respondents said they requested a drug. Not only are pharmaceutical companies pushing patients to act like consumers, but health insurance companies and politicians also see a way to reduce health care costs by viewing patients as consumers. In 2003, a Republican Congress introduced high-deductible plans. With these plans, subscribers pay for most health care services up to a certain amount ($5,800 for a single person and $11,600 for a family), and the insurance company covers most health care costs above that amount.[15] Typically, high-deductible plans cover one or two visits with a primary care physician for checkups, but they are essentially "catastrophic" insurance plans that cover only serious and expensive health events. To help individuals with high-deductible plans pay for health care, Congress passed a law that set up tax-exempt health saving accounts (HSA).[16] Individuals can "deposit" up to $3,000 per year to an HSA, and a family can deposit up to $5,950.[17] Money not spent in one year can be rolled over to the next year and can earn interest. In 2009, 12 percent of firms providing health insurance offered high-deductible health plans with HSAs.[18]

Supporters envisioned that such plans would reduce health care spending by turning patients into price-conscious consumers. Such consumers would shop for the highest quality of services at the lowest price, which would prompt physicians, hospitals, clinics, and laboratories to compete for patients by increasing efficiency. In this model, physicians are essentially seen as salespeople who *promote* certain products, such as surgeons who sell surgeries or primary care doctors who sell prescription orders and referrals. As with other salespeople, they provide information about the product they sell and may make recommendations, but ultimately the patient decides. This view of physicians is quite different from the traditional one of professionals *prescribing* treatment based on their comprehensive knowledge about medical conditions, knowledge they have acquired through years of medical training.

A reasonable question is whether patients-as-consumers will make decisions that result in better patient outcomes at lower costs. Patients typically are not very price sensitive. Consumers often use price as an indicator for quality when considering products and services that are not uniform and for which they do not have complete information. A discount surgeon is presumed to be cheaper because he provides a lower-quality product with worse patient outcomes—exactly the sort of surgeon patients would want to steer clear of.[19]

In 1963, more than a decade before health care became big business, Nobel Prize–winning economist Kenneth J. Arrow warned against further commercialization of health care. Arrow observed that the market for health care differs from that of other consumer goods. First, the demand for health care services is often irregular and unpredictable, and patients have limited knowledge about the services provided. Second, the supply of services is provided by professionals who have a monopoly over writing referrals to specialists, ordering diagnostic tests, and writing prescriptions. Because of these factors, the provision of services may not correspond to the actual demand of the "consumers." Finally, health care services differ from most other goods and services in that they are intrinsically tied to the consumers' well-being. In the case of life-threatening injury or illness, health care is essential for the survival of the consumer, and in such circumstances the consumer would be willing to pay anything for medical care. Arrow called the commercialization of health care an "assault on personal integrity."

Arrow concluded that because of the above-mentioned

differences between health care and other goods—including the gross asymmetry in information between the physician and the patient—competitive market forces cannot work, resulting in inefficient outcomes, specifically less health care at a higher cost.

The following story is an example of the problem of asymmetry of information and why it is impossible for patients to be consumers making good economic decisions. In 2005, my rheumatologist suggested that I see a physician who specialized in environmental medicine for my continued neurological problems, such as muscle twitching, migrating pains, and memory problems. The environmental physician speculated that I had become poisoned with pesticide during my childhood summer job as a strawberry picker at my grandfather's farm. I guess I may have been exposed to pesticide at an early age, but I don't remember having any ill effects from strawberry picking, other than an occasional achy stomach after eating too many strawberries.

The environmental physician did a thorough neurologic exam and recommended a series of blood tests for heavy metals and pesticides at a total cost of $1,800. The physician was in my health plan's network, but the laboratory was not. I asked to have the tests done by a laboratory covered by my plan, but the physician insisted that I have the tests done through his laboratory of choice. He explained that tests from other laboratories were of poor quality. He also told me that, in order for him to treat me, I would have to have a certain eye test with a price tag of $600 done at his office. As a patient with little knowledge about the long-term impact of toxins on the body, I could not determine whether these tests were, indeed, medically necessary. I had no way of knowing whether the laboratory the physician used was so much better than the laboratories covered by my insurance that it justified spending $1,800 instead of my copay of $10. I would have to believe that this physician was placing my best interests above his own monetary interests. I probably would have trusted the physician, since I am a risk-adverse patient. After all, if I needed these tests to uncover some hidden toxicological problem, they were my best hope for a complete recovery. In the end, the decision was rather straightforward: the physician had priced me out of the market. I simply did not have the money to pay for these tests.

Doctors' Conflict of Interest

The environmental doctor either owned or leased the eye-testing machine, and he made money every time he prescribed the test. Alternatively, a physician can earn a markup by ordering tests from a specific laboratory. A markup can take the form of a divergence between the price the physician charges the patient and what the laboratory is paid for running the tests. The physician may receive an excessive processing fee. One alternative medical practitioner I consulted charged $75 to draw blood. If, instead, she had written a requisition for the same tests to be done at my in-network laboratory, she would have earned nothing. Physicians can also make money from laboratory testing by investing in the specialized diagnostic laboratories they use.

Physicians' business ventures do not stop with the diagnostic testing industry. Cardiologists invest in artificial heart device companies, spinal surgeons invest in spinal device companies, and oncologists invest in pharmaceutical companies that develop new cancer drugs. An article in the *New York Times* described the increasingly close financial ties between spinal surgeons and start-up companies producing and selling spinal devices, such as screws.[20] In one case, 120 physicians each invested $50,000 or more in the California-based spinal device company Allez Spine

LLC. They then used the company's product on their patients. The nature of the investment agreement between physicians and the medical device company varies. Some physicians are "passive investors," whereas other physicians actively promote the products sold by the companies in which they invest. Investment agreements will often encourage physicians to be active investors by making the returns on the investment dependent on the investor physician's use of the company's product.

Moreover, it is not uncommon for medical researchers running clinical trials to have investments in the companies whose products they are testing. In a trial study on the effectiveness of an artificial spinal disk named Prodisk, physicians at eight of the seventeen research centers involved in the trial were invested in the company, Spinal Solutions, which had developed the spinal disk they were testing.[21] The trial study found Prodisk worked better than the traditional spinal fusion surgery and that the patients recovered more quickly. Based on these findings, the Food and Drug Administration (FDA) approved Prodisk, and the physician investors received great returns on their investment. Were the findings of the study compromised by the researchers' financial interests? Maybe. Of the 233 people who received the artificial disk, 50 patients were classified as "training cases," in which surgeons learned to perform the surgery, and they were not included in the final findings of the study. An additional 21 people were excluded due to unspecified reasons. If patients who fared poorly were excluded, the results of the trial would be skewed in favor of Prodisk.

Despite the fact that doctors' investments in companies that produce medical devices create a serious conflict of interest, the FDA does not prohibit physicians from investing in companies whose products they are testing, as long as they disclose to the government their financial ties. Disclosure to patients is not required, and the vast majority of patients remain in the dark about their doctors' investments.

One patient, Patricia Kennedy, had the Prodisk put in, but the surgery failed, and she ended up in even worse pain than before. She sued her spinal surgeon after learning that he had invested half a million dollars in Spinal Solutions, the company that had produced the spinal disk. The case was settled out of court on undisclosed terms.[22]

Another common relationship found between physicians and the investment industry involves the exchange of information about drug trials. Physicians are typically paid $300 to $500 per hour to talk to investors.[23] Approximately one in every ten physicians receive payment from investment companies, according to an article in the *Journal of American Medical Association*.[24] Insider information about drug trial outcomes can be very valuable for investment companies, as the drug companies' stock value can either skyrocket if a new drug is approved by the FDA or plummet if it is rejected.

In 2004, a new eye medication, Macugen, was approved by the FDA for the treatment of macular degeneration, which causes blindness. Macugen was produced by the small biotech company, Eyetech Pharmaceuticals. Soon after Macugen entered the market, another biotech company, Genentech, introduced the experimental drug Lucentis to treat the same eye condition. If the new experimental drug turned out to be more effective than Macugen, the stock values of both biotech companies would be greatly impacted. So Citigroup's large brokerage company, Smith Barney, set out to uncover how Lucentis fared in the drug trial compared to Macugen. Smith Barney did not fund new research to uncover new medical information. Instead, it paid 26 eye physicians involved in the government-funded drug trials to talk to them.[25]

Based on conversations with the physicians, Smith Barney determined that the experimental drug Lucentis was the superior drug. They issued a report on May 5, 2005, to select investors who may pay more than $1 million a year for this sort of information. Based on the information, insider-investors shorted the stock of Eyetech, which produced Macugen, in anticipation that the company's stock would fall in value. On May 23, Genentech, the producer of the superior experimental drug, publicly announced the findings of the comparative trial study. The findings were almost identical to the information obtained by Smith Barney. Eyetech's stock price plummeted to half its value, and the investors—with whom Citigroup had shared their insider information—earned 40 percent in return on their investment in less than three weeks. Other investors without the insider information saw their investment in Eyetech lose half its value.[26]

A small but increasing number of prominent academic scientists are severing their ties with pharmaceutical and medical device companies. Some physicians worry that their financial ties may subconsciously influence their judgment, while other physicians realize that such ties damage their credibility. One person who stopped accepting consulting fees is Dr. Eric P. Winer, director of the Breast Oncology Center at the Dana-Farber Cancer Institute at Harvard University. He said, "Several times when I was interviewed for stories, after my comment there would be the obligatory phase, 'Dr. Winer has accepted honoraria,' and I was tired of hearing that."[27]

In 2008, the Cleveland Clinic, one of the nation's leading medical research centers, began to publicly disclose doctors' industry ties. On their Web site, www.clevelandclinic.org, the

Cleveland Clinic lists consulting payments of more than $5,000 a year, and all royalty and equity interest in medical and pharmaceutical companies for each of its nearly 1,800 doctors on staff.[28] This sort of disclosure can be helpful in exposing potential conflicts of interest, but its accuracy still depends on physicians fully reporting their financial ties.

An investigation by the Republican senator Charles E. Grassley from Iowa revealed that universities and research hospitals do a poor job policing their doctors' conflicts of interest. Some argue that universities themselves have conflicts of interest because they also benefit from doctors' ties to the medical industry, in the form of hospital funding and prestige deriving from published research articles. The most egregious case was a psychiatrist, Dr. Charles B. Nemeroff, at Emory University in Atlanta, Georgia. Over a seven-year period, Dr. Nemeroff made at least $2.8 million from consulting deals with pharmaceutical companies.[29] In 2004, administrators at Emory University became concerned about potential conflicts of interest and requested that he limit his consulting fees to $10,000 a year. Dr. Nemeroff agreed to do so, but the next day he traveled to Jackson Hole, Wyoming, for a consulting gig paid for by the British pharmaceutical company GlaxoSmithKline Inc. Dr. Nemeroff stayed at the upscale Four Seasons resort and was paid $3,000 for his services in Jackson Hole. Before the year was over, Dr. Nemeroff had received a total of $170,000 in consulting fees from GlaxoSmithKline alone, all of which he kept secret from Emory University.

In 2007, Senator Grassley introduced legislation that would bring transparency into physicians' relationship with the medical industry. Provisions of the Physician Payments Sunshine Act of 2007 would have required pharmaceutical and medical device companies to publicly disclose their payments to physicians.[30]

Companies that failed to disclose such payments would have faced a penalty of $10,000 to $100,000. The bill did not outlaw consulting payments to doctors but required disclosure of doctors' conflicts of interest in their research on new drugs and medical devices, as well as in their medical practice. Such a law would undoubtedly cause more doctors to follow in the footsteps of Dr. Winer at Harvard University. [31]

Specialized Care

Advances in modern medicine have made the number of specialties grow into the hundreds, some so obscure that only those afflicted with a medical condition requiring their services ever even know they exist. From 1979 to 1999, the number of medical specialists per person increased by 118 percent, more than twice the rate of growth in the number of primary care physicians.[32] Almost two in every three physicians in the United States are specialists.[33] In comparison, only one in three physicians were specialists sixty years ago, and these specialized in only a few fields, such as general surgery, pediatrics, and gynecology.

At the same time, fewer students are entering the field of primary care. In 2007, only 7 percent of new graduates chose family practice, which has resulted in physician shortages, particularly in poorer rural regions.[34] A study by the Center for Health Policy Research at the Dartmouth Medical School in New Hampshire found that regions with shortages of primary care physicians had 36 percent fewer physicians for every 100,000 persons (after accounting for age and gender differences) than in high-supply regions.[35] Massachusetts mandated universal health coverage in 2007, which resulted in a sharp rise in the demand for primary care physicians. Despite being one of the leading medical centers in the world, Massachusetts faces a physician shortage.

The Massachusetts law requires all residents in the state to obtain health coverage. To increase access to affordable health insurance, most employers are required to offer it to their employees.[36] The state also offers subsidized plans to low-income people through a program called Commonwealth Care. An estimated 350,000 uninsured people have gained coverage since the law passed.[37] These previously uninsured people are lining up for checkups, and the waiting lists at primary care doctors are growing. [38]

Concern about a physician shortage is not new. In fact, the *New York Times* published a letter to the editor in 1919 with the headline "Failing Medical Schools; Shortage of Physicians Will Make Itself Felt a Few Years Hence." At the time, a big concern was that the country would soon face a doctor shortage because medical schools were closing down due to lack of funding. The problem was that medicine was not seen an attractive line of work for the well-off. As the *New York Times* piece noted: "Rich men's sons seldom study medicine—the work is too hard—the hours are too long—and the returns are not commensurate in a financial way with the effort."[39] So, mostly sons of less well-off families studied medicine, and most of them struggled to raise the money to pay for tuition, which was $250 (annually) at the time.

Today, the cost of education is also a problem. Average annual tuition and fees at a state medical school were $23,581 for in-state residents and $43,587 for nonresidents in 2008–09.[40] Most medical students leave medical school with substantial debt. Fifty percent graduate with a debt of more than $155,000, so the fact that many medical students seek specialties that pay well is not surprising. The combination of high tuition along with the skewed reimbursement structure of insurance plans discourages medical students from becoming primary care physicians. According to data from the Medical Group Management Association, dermatologists earned a median annual income of $368,400 in 2000.[41] Orthopedic surgeons had the highest median annual income, just short of $500,000. Primary care physicians, on the other hand, earned a median annual income of $186,000.

The increasing reliance on specialists has driven up health care costs. Americans spent $509 billion on physicians and clinical services (not including hospitals) in 2008, or $1,669 per person.[42] And expenditures on physicians are rising rapidly—up 50 percent from the beginning of the decade. The number of practicing physicians is not higher in the United States than it is in Europe.[43] However, Americans rely more heavily on specialists for care, and American physicians rely more heavily on technology in the screening, diagnosis, and monitoring of diseases than do their European counterparts. For instance, the number of magnetic resonance imaging (MRI) machines and computed tomography (CT) scanners in the United States is substantially higher than in Europe (see table 3.1).

In the United States, it is increasingly common for specialists to acquire CT scanners and MRI units for their own practice, leading to both underutilization and overuse. On-site scanners are convenient for both the patient and the physician and reduce the time of diagnosis, but they also give the physician a financial incentive to overprescribe tests. To address this conflict of interest, Congress passed the Stark Law in 1992, prohibiting physicians from referring Medicare patients to the physician's own scanning devices. However, a loophole in the law exempts on-site scanners, effectively negating the regulation. The loophole allows a cardiologist who has

TABLE 3.1 Number of practicing physicians, MRI units, and CT scanners in the United States, Canada, and selected European countries, 2007

	# of practicing physicians (per 1000 population)	# of MRI units (per 100,000 population)	# of CT scanners (per 100,000 population)	Health expenditures (per person in US$ PPP)
United States	2.4	25.9	34.3	$7,290
Belgium	4.0	7.5	41.6	3,595
Canada	2.2	6.7	12.7	3,895
France	3.4	5.7	10.3	3,601
Germany	3.5	8.2	16.3	3,588
United Kingdom	2.5	8.2	7.6	2,992

Source: OECD 2009.
Note: Purchasing power parity (PPP) is a currency conversion rate that both converts a foreign currency into U.S. dollars and adjusts for cost-of-living.

invested in a $1 million CT scanner to self-refer patients without restrictions. CT angiograms typically cost $500–$1500—or about ten times that of X-ray angiograms. So CT scans are driving up health care costs even though there is little scientific evidence showing that they are significantly better in diagnosing and monitoring heart disease.[44] They may, in fact, harm patients in the long run. CT scanners expose patients to much higher levels of radiation per scan—about 100 times more than X-ray machines—thereby increasing patients' risk of cancer from radiation exposure.

Unaffordable Care

Physicians increasingly operate as for-profit businesses, not unlike publicly traded corporations. More and more physicians have a financial stake in specialized diagnostic laboratories from which they order tests. They own shares in medical companies that

BOX 3
How to Find a Good Doctor

1. Word of mouth: Ask friends, neighbors, coworkers, and family about their doctors. When looking for a primary care physician, make sure that the physician listens to the patient, answers questions, returns phone calls, and has a friendly office staff. When seeking a specialist, look for one who has extensive experience in treating your particular medical condition. One way to meet patients with the same medical problem is to attend local patient support-group meetings.

2. Recommendation: If looking for a specialist, ask your primary care physician. But keep in mind that your primary care physician might have a business relationship with a specific medical facility or hospital and is likely to recommend specialists affiliated with that facility or hospital, even if the specialists are not necessarily the best in your area.

3. The Internet: Look for doctor recommendations and ratings on the Internet. You can read other patients' ratings of doctors on Web sites such as: www.doctorscorecard.com, www.rateMDs.com, www.mydochub.com, and www.drscore.com. You can find information about how well hospitals care for their patients at the government Web site, www.hospitalcompare.hhs.gov.

3. Top doctors: A specialist at a research hospital is more likely to be up on the latest research and conduct research on new

treatments. But leading researchers also have their downside. Research physicians may not have good bedside manners. They might not take the time to listen to the patient, and they can be difficult to reach in case of a medical emergency. Research physicians are more likely to travel to attend conferences and consulting events. Finally, research physicians are more likely to have financial arrangements with pharmaceutical and medical device companies, which could create a conflict of interest.

4. Background check: Check with your state medical board to find out if a physician has been disciplined, sued for malpractice, or is currently being investigated by the board of medicine. This information can be obtained from the medical board's Web site in your state.

5. Meet-and-greet consultation: Schedule a consultation with a physician before handing over your care to that person. Ask how many cases similar to yours the physician has treated. Some insurance plans do not cover such consultations, but if you can afford the fee, it may be well worth it, especially in the case of a complicated medical condition.

6. Warning: Beware of hospitals, medical clinics, and physicians who advertise on television, radio, and magazines. If they were as great as they claim, they would likely have plenty of patients and would not need to advertise for new patients.

produce the medical devices they use, and they hold patents on pharmaceutical products. This entanglement of financial interests with the practice of medicine creates a fundamental conflict of interest, in which patients may receive inferior medical care at a higher cost. The end result is that health care in the United States is much more expensive than it needs to be.

Americans pay on average twice as much for health care as people do in France, Germany, and the United Kingdom. The difference between the United States and Europe is even more striking when one considers that these European countries all have universal coverage, while 42 percent of all working-age Americans are either uninsured or underinsured.[45] Moreover, health care costs are rising faster in the United States, further increasing the spending gap between the United States and Europe.

Health care in the United States has become highly stratified, where people with good insurance coverage or the financial means to pay, can obtain top care. This minority of Americans, which includes business leaders, politicians, and professionals, has access to leading specialists, can undergo sophisticated diagnostic testing and cutting-edge medical procedures, and can afford to fill prescriptions for the newest and most expensive drugs available. For this group of people, the current health care system is working pretty well. However, the majority of the population does not have access to this type of care, even if they have insurance coverage. Top-notch health care by leading specialists is far out of reach for the vast majority of underinsured patients.

Of course, European publicly funded health care also has shortcomings. Waiting lists for nonemergency conditions, such as cataracts of the eye, are not uncommon in most European countries. But the U.S. health care system also has rationing. Here rationing takes on a different form and is enacted through pricing. People who have insurance that does not cover their medical needs, or who do not have insurance at all, will have to forgo treatment if they cannot afford to pay for the treatment out of pocket. Like patients in Europe, these individuals are on a "waiting list" for treatment, but unlike European patients, they may wait indefinitely . . . or until their financial status improves.

FOUR

Drugs

QUANTITY OVERRIDE

I HAD ALREADY BEEN SICK FOR THREE YEARS when I arrived at my endocrinologist's office for a follow-up appointment after developing a hyperactive thyroid problem. As I entered the waiting room five minutes before my scheduled appointment time, I noticed that every single seat was taken, but there was only one other patient. The rest of the people were sales representatives from various pharmaceutical companies. They sat there with their little black suitcases filled with free drug samples, pens, and paper pads, chatting it up as if they were attending a cocktail party. Engagement rings and wedding planning were popular topics among female sales reps, while their male counterparts stuck with less personal topics, such as sports and the latest TV shows. I slid a pile of magazines away from a corner of the coffee table and settled in for what turned out to be a 45-minute wait. I then waited in the exam room for an additional 15 minutes. During this wait, I couldn't help overhearing the doctor chatting with two sales reps about golfing in Florida.

Free Samples

The ubiquitous sales reps are increasingly crowding doctors' offices and crowding out doctors' time with patients. In a decade, the number of sales reps increased from 56,000 to 88,000.[1] In comparison, there are about 800,000 practicing physicians in the United States. With more of them competing for busy physicians' time, sales reps have become increasingly innovative in getting the doctor's attention. Some salespeople will bring gifts, such as tickets to sporting events. Some will run errands for the doctor, such as picking up a cup of coffee on the way. Much attention is paid to appearance. Sales reps wear stylish clothes. Women have impeccably styled hair, and their makeup is never smudged. Some female sales reps have been observed wearing unseemly short skirts when visiting male doctors, enduring below-freezing temperatures in the winter and bone-chilling air blasting from the air conditioner in the summer. Whatever the method, the main goal of drug salespeople is to promote prescription drugs sold by their pharmaceutical companies.

The drugs they promote are the newest and more expensive brand-name drugs, and the role of a sales rep is to "educate" the doctor about the benefits of the drug. Salespeople will provide the doctor with data, collected by the pharmaceutical companies, showing that their drugs are more effective and have fewer side effects than competing drugs. In the case of a busy family doctor with a waiting room full of patients, sales reps are often the sole source of information that the doctor receives about the drug.[2]

But sales representatives may not be the best source of information. They rarely have college degrees in chemistry or a related science. Rather, an increasing number of drug reps are former cheerleaders.[3] Cheerleaders make good salespeople because they are attractive, cheerful, and friendly, but they are not experts on pharmaceuticals. A 1995 study found that 11 percent of sales reps' statements were incorrect, and all the incorrect claims were skewed in favor of the drug they were promoting.[4] Howard Brody, a physician with the Center for Ethics and Humanities in the Life Sciences, would like physicians to refuse to see sales reps altogether. After all, given the inaccuracy of information provided by sales reps, a physician would still have to do independent research on these new drugs; such research would be a more efficient use of doctors' time than listening to sales pitches.

In addition to information, sales reps bring doctors gifts. They are often seen trucking along a small suitcase filled with free drug samples. The distribution of samples is an integral part of drug promotion by sales reps. Free drug samples allow the doctor to try out a new medication without the patient incurring any costs. For patients with limited or no health insurance, the value of free samples can translate into hundreds of dollars saved. The Lyme disease specialist I am currently seeing is a very nice person, and it pains him to give patients bad news. To compensate for the bad news, he gives out free samples. The worse the news, the bigger the bag of free samples I take home with me. On the other hand, if the doctor has good news, the patient often leaves empty-handed. Like my Lyme disease doctor, many doctors use free samples as a gift-giving gesture to make the patients feel good about the consultation or appease them at time of payment.

However, free samples are not the win-win situation they may seem to be, one that allows patients to try out a new drug for free and pharmaceutical companies to promote their newest medication. Free drug samples can also influence physicians' medical judgment. *Consumer Reports* specifically warns patients against accepting free samples because "they might not be the best choice."[5] A study of family practitioners in four medical clinics found that physicians who dispersed free samples also wrote more prescriptions for these drugs.[6] Even in the case where a preferred alternative was available, physicians were still more likely to prescribe the drugs for which they had received free samples. Moreover, when physicians stop receiving free samples of a drug, they prescribe less of the drug. A *New York Times* article quotes a study that found that physicians' use of first-line drugs (as recommended by national guidelines) to treat patients with hypertension increased sharply after free drug samples for alternative hypertension drugs were removed.[7]

Moreover, free samples are not exactly free, as patients and their insurance companies end up paying for them when patients fill their prescription. Drug companies distribute free drug samples to promote their latest and most expensive brand-name drugs. If free samples were available for cheaper alternatives, doctors would be more likely to prescribe these. In her book, *The Big Fix*, Katharine Greider describes an initiative to encourage doctors to prescribe cheaper generic drugs.[8] A national insurance company joined forces with a large pharmaceutical company to offer 1,700 physicians from across the country free samples of selected generic drugs. Eighteen months later, prescriptions for these drugs had increased by 22 percent. This suggests that doctors are more likely to put patients on a medication simply because they have free samples in their medicine cabinet and not because they are necessarily the superior drug.

Gift Giving

Sample medicines are not the only gift that sales representatives hand out when they visit doctors. Pens, note pads, and posters with the pharmaceutical company logo litter surfaces and walls of most doctors' offices. Prescription pads printed with the pharmaceutical company's name stare in the face of doctors when it is time to write a prescription. Under U.S. law, it is illegal for pharmaceutical companies to pay doctors to prescribe their medication, but in-kind gifts are almost entirely unregulated. For instance, it is illegal for a pharmaceutical company to offer money to physicians, but it is not illegal to reimburse physicians for expenses incurred while attending a medical conference.

A survey of patient awareness and approval of gifts from pharmaceutical companies to physicians found high awareness of some gifts, such as free samples of drugs, but low awareness of other types of gifts, such as restaurant dinners.[9] Patients were split in their attitudes about gift giving by pharmaceutical companies. Almost half of patients surveyed thought that dinner at a restaurant was inappropriate for doctors to accept. Interestingly, approval rates were fairly high for gifts considered to be trivial or that had potential value to patient care. For instance, less than 8 percent of patients disapproved of free drug samples.

Most patients are generally unaware that common practices in academic medical centers can cause a conflict of interest for physicians. Such practices include the following:

1. physicians participating in pharmaceutical companies' speaker bureaus;
2. physicians publishing articles that were ghostwritten by pharmaceutical industry officials;
3. physicians serving on panels that recommend which drugs should be prescribed, while having financial ties with one or more drug companies;

4. pharmaceutical companies paying for physicians' continu-
    ing education classes, which are often held at desirable
    locations, such as Hawaii;

5. pharmaceutical companies reimbursing medical students
    for their textbooks.

One of the arguably more unethical promotional strategies
adopted by pharmaceutical companies in recent years is "seeding
trials." One pharmaceutical company paid 2,500 Maryland physicians for participating in a drug trial of its new blood-pressure medicine.[10] Each physician was paid $1,050 to enroll twelve patients
in the trial. The drug trial had the appearance of being a research
project, but no information of interest was collected. Instead, the
purpose of such seeding trials is to promote a new drug by paying
physicians for prescribing the drug to their patients. By the end
of the "trial study," the physician has gained experience using the
drug and is more likely to continue to prescribe it. But seeding
trials essentially allow pharmaceutical companies to evade the law
that prohibits direct payments to physicians for prescribing their
drugs. Moreover, such trials fundamentally undermine the trust
between a doctor and the patient, for, under the false pretext of
research, the physician receives a financial incentive to prescribe
a medication that is not necessarily the preferable medication.[11]

In 2005, the pharmaceutical industry spent about $25 billion
to promote drugs to physicians and an additional $4.2 billion
in advertisements directed at consumers.[12] In comparison, U.S.
pharmaceutical companies spent about $20 billion on the research
and development of new drugs.[13] This aggressive promotion of
drugs is influencing doctors' prescription patterns by increasing
prescriptions for expensive brand-name medicines that may not

necessarily be the preferred drug. The end result is that patients are paying more and getting less for their money.

Patents, Pills, and Patients

Pharmaceutical companies spend billions of dollars each year to promote their brand-name drugs because they are in a race against time to sell as many pills as possible before the patent expires. The federal government grants pharmaceutical patents for 20 years, making the patent holder the exclusive producer of the patented drug for that length of time. The reasoning behind a patent is that for its duration the pharmaceutical company can charge monopoly price—well above the market price—for the drug to recover research and development (R&D) expenditures.

After the patent expires, other pharmaceutical companies can produce the same drug and market it under its generic name. Generic drugs are bio-equivalent to the original brand-name drug: they have the same composition of active ingredients and the exact same properties, although the inactive ingredients may vary. For instance, the color, size, and shape of generic drugs may differ from the brand-name drug. A study by the Food and Drug Administration (FDA) found that the price of a drug drops 6 percent, on average, after the first generic enters the market, but a full 50 percent after the second generic enters the market.[14] By the time the sixth generic becomes available, the price has dropped 75 percent.

Pharmaceutical companies employ several methods to delay the entrance of competing generics on the market. One such strategy is to sue the generic firm for patent infringement. The brand-name manufacturer will often not be successful in its case, but the suit will delay the introduction of the generic. According to a 2002 report by the Federal Trade Commission (FTC), brand-name companies win only about one quarter of their patent infringement cases decided in court.[15] But under the Drug Price Competition and Patent Restoration Act of 1984, or the Hatch-Waxman Act for short, the FDA cannot approve a generic drug for 30 months or until litigation is settled if the brand-name manufacturer contests a generic based on patent infringement.

An estimated 110 brand-name drugs, with total sales revenue of $50 billion per year, will lose their patents between 2007 and 2010.[16] This is equal to average revenues of $1.2 million per drug per day for pills that cost only a few cents each to produce. This means that the brand-name manufacturer makes over a million dollars in sales for every day it can delay the introduction of a generic. For some drugs, the gain is even greater. Therefore, brand-name companies are willing to pay large sums of money to a generic manufacturer to delay the introduction of a generic. The FTC found that 7 out of every 10 settlements of patent infringement cases included a payment from the brand-name company to the generic company in exchange for deferred entry of the generic.[17]

Alternatively, a brand-name company can introduce its own "authorized generic." Under the Hatch-Waxman Act, the first company that submits an application to produce a generic is granted a 6-month exclusivity to market the generic. The purpose of this provision is to encourage generic manufacturers to enter the market despite the threat of litigation from the brand-name manufacturer by giving them the exclusive right to produce and sell the generic for a limited period of time. During this period, they can charge a higher than normal price because they share the market only with the brand-name drug. In the case of an authorized generic, the brand-name manufacturer will typically enter into an agreement with a generic company (sometimes its own subsidiary) that gives the partner company the right to produce the generic under the brand-name drug's patent, without facing litigation, in exchange for payment.[18]

One example of an authorized generic is azithromycin, the generic of Zithromax. Azithromycin is one of the most commonly prescribed antibiotics in the world, used to treat a long list of infections, including Lyme disease. In 2005, Pfizer Inc., the manufacturer of brand-name Zithromax, earned about $2 billion in sales revenues on the drug.[19] When the patent for Zithromax expired in November of that year, Pfizer launched a generic version of the drug through its own subsidiary, Greenstone Inc., to immediately capture the new generic market. In addition, Pfizer filed a "citizen petition" with the FDA claiming that two other generic manufacturers did not accurately label the active ingredients in the drug and asking the FDA to recall the mislabeled generics. Pfizer also took legal action claiming patent infringement against the generic manufacturers. The FDA did not recall the generics in question, and Pfizer subsequently settled its patent case for an undisclosed amount. The year following the expiration of its patents, Pfizer's worldwide sales revenues dropped 68 percent to $638 million. In 2004, a prescription of 40 pills (600 mg) of the brand-name Zithromax cost $378. By December 2007, the price had fallen to $299 for the generic azithromycin.[20]

Rather than challenge the introduction of a generic in court, the brand-name company can instead preempt the launch of the generic by developing a reformulated version of the drug. Before the patent expires, the brand-name manufacturer may take out a

new patent for a slightly different version of the drug. Reformula-
tion of a drug could be a change in delivery mechanism, such as a
slow release form to make the effect of the medication last longer,
or the change of a pill to a fluid or a spray. Usually, the brand-name
company will aggressively promote the reformulated drug to physicians and consumers through advertisement and distribution of
free samples.

One such case is Ambien, a popular sleep medication. Before
the patent for Ambien expired in April 2007, Sanofi-aventis, the
manufacturer of Ambien, developed a new version of the drug,
Ambien CR. "CR" stands for "controlled release." The new pill
consists of two layers of active ingredients; the second layer is a
slow release, making the drug work throughout the night. Sanofi-
aventis launched Ambien CR in October 2005 with a broad
advertisement campaign on television and full-page spreads in
magazines and newspapers. The ads showed happy people sleeping and offered seven-day free trial coupons of the medication.[21]
Sanofi-aventis was successful in shifting demand to their new
reformulated drug before their patent for the old version expired,
thereby making the generic for the old version almost obsolete.
Increasingly, R&D money is directed toward developing reformulated drugs rather than new drugs.

A study by the National Institute of Health Care Management (NIHCM) found that fully 65 percent of drugs approved
by the FDA were "product-line extensions," which used old ingredients, and only 35 percent contained new active ingredients.[22]
Furthermore, less than half of the drugs containing new active
ingredients were deemed by the FDA to provide a significant
improvement. All in all, the NIHCM estimates that only 15 percent of new drugs approved contain new active ingredients and
are significantly better than existing drugs on the market.

Restrictions

The introduction of new and expensive drugs, which are not necessarily better and often not much different from drugs already available, has made the cost of drugs rise rapidly. The Centers for Medicare and Medicaid Services (CMS) projects that Americans will spend a total of $245 billion on prescription drugs in 2009.[23] Moreover, expenditures per person on prescription drugs have been increasing at an annual rate of 5.3 percent—more that double the rate of inflation.

Because of rising drug prices, insurance companies make patients jump through hoops to fill a prescription. The following story actually happened to me in 2004 and got repeated on a regular basis throughout my illness: I arrive at my local pharmacy with a new prescription. I am told that the pharmacy doesn't have the medication in stock and that I will have to come back the next day after noon. The following afternoon I return only to learn that the medication was not delivered, and I should come back the following day. The following day, I call the pharmacy to make sure that they have received the medication. It is there, so I make yet another trip to the pharmacy, only to discover that the charge is $380. The pharmacist tells me that my health plan does not cover the medication. I leave the medication there and go home to call my health plan. The service representative tells me that the medication requires pre-authorization. I call my doctor to ask her to request pre-authorization. No one at the doctor's office picks up the phone, so I leave a message. The next day, the doctor's receptionist calls me back and tells me that I need to fax them the pre-authorization form. I call my health plan again to have them fax the doctor the pre-authorization form. The service representative refers me to the health plan's pharmacist, who tells me that I don't need pre-authorization; instead, my doctor needs to call in a notification. I call the doctor's office again to ask them to call in the notification. I wait two days before I venture down to the pharmacy again. On my fourth trip, I am in luck and I get my prescription for the cost of my copay.

Health insurance companies regularly require patients to obtain doctor notification and pre-authorization, and they place other restrictions on prescription drug coverage. A restriction on the quantity of pills covered by insurance is common. My health plan has placed quantity restrictions on about 25 percent of covered prescription drugs.[24] For some prescription drugs, I can fill only a 10-days supply of medication at a time, meaning that I have to make three trips in one month to fill a month's worth of medication and pay my copay three times. My plan covers only 10 out of every 30 days of other drugs, leaving me to pay for the remaining 20 days or experience long breaks in my medication. For antibiotics, such a gap in treatment is a well-known way to create treatment-resistant bacteria.

Faced with the choice of forgoing my doctor-prescribed medical treatment or shelling out hundreds of dollars on the antibiotic cefdinir (the generic of Omnicef), I called my insurance plan's pharmacist for advice. At first, the insurance pharmacist refused to make any recommendation about my treatment. After repeatedly pressuring her to advise me about the numbers of days I should take the medication—the amount covered by my insurance plan or the amount prescribed by my physician—she finally suggested that I request a "quantity override" from my pharmacist.

I had never heard about a quantity override before. It turns out that in the case of a restriction on the quantity of a prescription drug, my pharmacy can ask for an override. I just have to say the two magic words, "quantity override," and my insurance plan lifts its restriction on the number of pills. By the time I first learned about quantity override, I had already been undergoing treatment for almost four years and had paid out thousands of dollars for medications not fully covered by my insurance plan. In those four years, my local pharmacist had never asked for an override on my behalf. I suspect that my pharmacy has a financial interest in having me rather than my insurance plan pay for prescription drugs: insurance companies pay a lower price than customers who pay directly for prescription medication.

For those of us who are very sick and need prescription medication the most, penetrating the maze of rules and requirements is almost impossible. Insurance companies take advantage of these difficulties and effectively limit prescription coverage for us. As a result, we are more likely to end up paying for drugs out of pocket.

Drug Shopping

When your insurance coverage will not pay for a prescription drug, do some price shopping before filling a prescription, as pharmacies charge very different prices for the same drug. I conducted a small survey of pharmacies in and around Washington DC. I called 12 pharmacies and asked how much it would cost me to fill a month's prescription for Celebrex, a popular arthritis medication (60 capsules of 200 mg each). I chose Celebrex because it is a commonly prescribed brand-name drug that was aggressively promoted by Pfizer when it first entered the market in 1998 (the TV ads included an adorable border collie that did yoga). I soon discovered that prices varied substantially from one pharmacy to another. The most expensive pharmacy in Washington DC was CVS (at Dupont

TABLE 4.1 Price for a prescription of Celebrex
(60 capsules of 200 mg) in Washington DC;
Gaithersburg, MD; and Fairfax, VA, December 2007

Pharmacy Name	Location		Price
CVS	DC	Dupont Circle	$258.99
Safeway	DC	Adams Morgan	$247.00
Tschiffery Pharmacy	DC	Duport Circle	$244.74
CVS	DC	Anacostia	$241.99
Rite Aid	DC	Adams Morgan	$239.98
Rite Aid	VA	Fairfax	$243.99
CVS	MD	Gaithersburg	$241.99
CVS	VA	Fairfax	$241.99
Wal-Mart	VA	Fairfax	$213.84
Sam's Club	MD	Gaithersburg	$184.68

Circle), which charged $258.99 for Celebrex. The cheapest phar-
macy I contacted in the District of Columbia was RiteAid, which
sold Celebrex for 8 percent less, at $239.98 (see table 4.1).

One can find significant savings in the suburbs. CVS charged
lower prices in the suburbs than in the city, and discount pharmacies charged even less. The lowest price I found for Celebrex
was a shocking 40 percent below the price of one of the CVS
stores in DC. Sam's Club, located about a 30-minute drive north
in Gaithersburg, Maryland, charged only $184.68 for a month's
worth of Celebrex, and I was told that I don't even need to be a
Sam's Club member. But, in order to take advantage of the lower
prices in discount pharmacies, one has to have the health and
means to get there. Many elderly people residing in Washington
DC do not own a car or may not be able to drive due to a medical
condition. This is exactly why city pharmacies can charge higher
prices than pharmacies in the suburbs, despite the fact that their
customers often are less financially well-off.

Drug Importation

Another place to buy cheap drugs is Canada, but buying drugs outside the United States happens to be illegal. Under the Prescription Drug Marketing Act of 1988, anyone other than the drug's original manufacturer is prohibited from importing a prescription drug into the United States, though individuals can carry back to the United States small amounts of prescription drugs (less than three months' worth) for personal use. Over the first decade of the 21st century as the discrepancy between the prices of brand-name drugs sold in the United States and Canada has grown, more people have been traveling to Canada to fill their prescriptions.

As public pressure mounted to legalize the importation of prescription drugs, the pharmaceutical industry fought back, arguing that imported medications are unsafe for consumers. Former U.S. House Representative Billy Tauzin, now the president and CEO of the Pharmaceutical Research and Manufacturers of America (PhRMA), testified to Congress that "legalizing the importation of prescription drugs from foreign countries could threaten patient safety and also impact the future innovations of life-saving medications."[25] Such testimony gives the impression that prescription drugs sold in the United States are produced in the United States under rigorous oversight of the FDA and that drugs imported from Canada and Europe do not fall under FDA inspection, and are therefore unsafe.

So, I was surprised to discover that one of my medications, Mepron, to treat babesiosis, had "made in Canada" printed on it. Mepron is a thick, bright-yellow liquid that looks like paint and also tastes like it. It is a brand-name drug that costs almost its weight in gold. A bottle of Mepron, containing 210 milliliters (less than a cup) provides 21 days of medication and costs $1117 at my local pharmacy. Though the drug is made in Canada, I cannot legally buy it in Canada.

I then took a closer look at other medications in my medicine cabinet. Free samples and other packaged medications sometimes list the manufacturing location. I discovered that my migraine medication, Maxalt, is produced in England, and fluconazole (generic of the anti-yeast medication Diflucan) is made in India. Celebrex is produced in the United States on the island of Puerto Rico. Puerto Rico became the preferred location of many U.S. drug companies in the 1960s, when tax incentives made the island one of the world's leading global drug-making centers. Pharmaceutical companies on the island employ around 30,000 workers; drugs account for a quarter of Puerto Rican gross domestic product (GDP) and represent 60 percent of the island's exports.[26]

The reality is that most prescription drugs purchased in the United States are not produced in the United States. A 2007 study by the U.S. Government Accountability Office (GAO), the investigative arm of Congress, identified 3,249 foreign pharmaceutical manufacturers from all corners of the world that produce medicine for the U.S. market.[27] India and China are hot spots for pharmaceutical production and had the largest number of facilities, followed by Canada. In Africa, facilities manufacturing drugs for the U.S. market can be found in the countries of Democratic Republic of the Congo, Nigeria, Kenya, and South Africa. But it is unlikely you'll find "Made in Democratic Republic of the Congo" on your medication bottle, as this is information the pharmaceutical companies do not like to advertise.

The GAO estimates that only 60 percent of drugs sold in the

United States are produced in the United States (including Puerto Rico). Moreover, many of the drugs produced in the United States use active ingredients produced elsewhere. Overall, 80 percent of active ingredients used to make drugs sold in the United States are imported.

Should consumers be concerned about foreign-produced drugs? It depends. Pharmaceutical facilities located in Canada and Europe likely have the same standards of safety and control as U.S. facilities and may have even higher standards. Moreover, both domestic and foreign facilities are subject to inspections by the FDA.

But outside Europe and Canada, FDA inspections of foreign facilities fall short. The FDA relies on domestic staff to volunteer for foreign inspections. Not surprisingly, some locations are more attractive than others, and the FDA expended much of its resources on inspections of European facilities. In 2007, 24 inspections took place in France, 22 in Germany, 19 in Italy, 14 in Switzerland, and 13 in the United Kingdom. China received 13 inspections, but it has almost seven times more registered pharmaceutical establishments than the United Kingdom and has significantly laxer enforcement of safety standards than other countries.

According to an investigation by the GAO, the FDA cannot determine whether it has ever inspected 2,133 of the 3,249 registered foreign facilities.[28] Moreover, the FDA does an even worse job of keeping track of unregistered facilities. The GAO noted that the FDA does not know how many foreign establishments are subject to inspection, but estimates the number could be as high as 6,800 facilities.[29] This weak FDA oversight outside Canada and Europe creates an incentive for drug manufacturers to invest in production facilities in China and other such places.

In Puerto Rico, plants have closed down after FDA inspectors found issues with quality control. Rather than improving quality at those facilities, the companies decided to relocate. Over an 18-month period in 2006–07, the closure of five pharmaceutical plants in Puerto Rico meant the loss of more than 3,000 jobs.[30]

The proliferation of internationally produced drugs—drugs developed by a U.S. pharmaceutical company and produced in country X with active ingredients from countries Y and Z—makes it increasingly difficult for the FDA and consumers to track where, and by whom, active ingredients are actually produced. Consumers can only hope that pharmaceutical companies will set high standards for their suppliers and take upon themselves the responsibility to inspect foreign facilities. Pharmaceutical companies have a strong monetary incentive to do so; class action suits brought by patients who get sick or don't get better due to defective medication can be devastatingly expensive. On the other hand, if a mishap were to happen, a pharmaceutical company may find that covering it up, rather than warning the public, is in its best interest.

This is exactly what happened in the case of contamination of heparin, a blood-thinning drug used in cardiac surgery and kidney dialysis. The first reported cases of allergic reactions to heparin showed up in November 2007. But it took more than three months, four documented deaths, and 350 cases of severe allergic reactions before the drug was finally withdrawn from the market.[31] The problematic heparin was distributed by the large drug company Baxter International, but the drug itself was manufactured by the Wisconsin-based Scientific Protein Laboratory (SPL), which operated two plants, one in the United States and the other in China. Investigation by the FDA determined that the contaminated drug came from the Chinese plant. The Chinese plant in Changzhou city opened in 2004 but had never been inspected by the FDA.[32] Baxter International had filed the proper paperwork with the FDA, but the FDA confused the Changzhou SPL company with another pharmaceutical company with a similar name, and inspected that plant instead.[33] Chinese authorities also didn't inspect the Changzhou SPL plant because they only inspect pharmaceutical facilities, and the Changzhou SPL plant was considered a chemical facility.

But contaminated heparin was not confined to the Changzhou SPL plant alone. Soon, cases of severe allergic reactions were reported in Germany as well. The German heparin was produced at a different Chinese plant. Contaminated heparin originating from 12 Chinese plants was eventually identified in 10 other countries.[34] Further investigation by the FDA uncovered that the heparin was contaminated with chondroitin sulfate, a dietary supplement used for joint pain. In some batches of heparin, the contaminant made up as much as 50 percent.[35] The active ingredient of heparin is made from an enzyme extracted from the mucous membranes in pig intestines. Pig farmers sell the pig intestines to local family workshops that mix and cook the membranes. The unregulated workshops sell the processed membranes to middlemen, called consolidators, who then sell it to chemical plants, like the Changzhou SPL plant. Chondroitin sulfate, on the other hand, is produced from pig cartilage and in an over-sulfated form has the same blood-thinning properties as heparin. Because both heparin and chondroitin sulfate are derived from pigs, the contamination was not detected by the FDA's standard quality control testing when the product crossed the border into the United States.

Chondroitin sulfate is much cheaper to produce—about a twentieth of the cost of heparin. The chondroitin sulfate was

BOX 4

How to Reduce the Costs of Prescription Drugs

The high cost of prescription drugs is an obstacle for many patients. Patients often skip pills or break pills in half because they cannot afford their medications. For patients without drug coverage, filling prescriptions is expensive. Even patients with drug coverage may have to pay hundreds of dollars due to high copayments, stringent preapproval rules, and restrictions on duration of treatment or the quantity of pills covered under the plan.

1. Ask your doctor for a cheaper alternative. The latest brand-name drug may not necessarily be more effective in treating your medical condition. If you cannot afford the medication prescribed, tell your doctor.

2. If a generic version of the brand-name drug has been approved by the FDA, ask for the generic. The generic is bio-equivalent to the brand-name drug, meaning it has the same active ingredients and delivery mechanism.

3. Older generations of drugs may be as effective, and sometimes better, than newer drugs. The FDA has no requirements that new drugs be superior to older generations of drugs to be approved. New drugs may also have unknown side effects that show up only after several years of usage.

4. If you don't have drug coverage, you can realize substantial savings by price shopping. Prices vary substantially across pharmacies. Discount pharmacies—such as Wal-Mart, Sam's Club, and Costco—will generally charge lower prices.

5. Buy large quantities of medication that you expect to take over a longer period of time.

6. If you are a member of AAA (American Automobile Association) you can get an average discount of 15 percent off brand-name drugs and 35 percent off generics if you don't have insurance coverage or your insurance does not cover a specific drug. The size of the discount varies by pharmacy and drug, and not all drugs are covered. To claim the discount, go to www.aaa.com/prescriptions, and print out a "prescription savings card" to show along with your AAA card at your pharmacy. Most pharmacies accept the AAA discount.

7. Brand-name drugs are substantially cheaper in Canada. But beware of online pharmacies that claim to be Canadian. Verify independently that they are really selling and shipping prescription drugs from Canada. The state of Minnesota operates a Web site from which Americans can order medication from a list of Canadian pharmacies (www.state.mn.us/portal/mn/jsp/home.do?agency=Rx). Purchasing drugs through this Web site assures that the drugs are, in fact, from Canada.

8. Most pharmaceutical companies have patient-assistance programs that provide prescription medication at a reduced price or for free to low-income people without drug coverage. Partnership for Prescription Assistance (www.pparx .org) provides information and links to about 475 prescription programs offered by pharmaceutical companies, health companies, nonprofit organizations, and public programs.

9. State and local governments offer low-cost prescription programs for low-income, elderly, and uninsured people. To find out more about such programs in your area, contact your state or county health department.

added as a cheap filler at some point in the supply chain. However, its high sulfate content causes allergic reactions in people with sulfate allergies. This long chain—from pig farmers to unregulated family workshops, to various middlemen, to the Changzhou SPL plant that manufactured the drug, to the parent company in Wisconsin that sold it to Baxter International, that finalized the vials at a New Jersey plant and sold them to hospitals and dialysis centers—provides plenty of opportunities for contamination. When the FDA finally inspected the Changzhou SPL plant in February 2008, they uncovered irregularities at the plant and found that some heparin was made from "material from an unacceptable workshop vendor."[36] A spokeswoman with Baxter International further disclosed to the *New York Times* that "Baxter's investigators had been denied access to the consolidators and workshop" and therefore these were never inspected.[37]

In 2007, a pig virus swept across China killing millions of pigs and making pig intestines less readily available. The shortage of intestines may have contributed to the problem of drug contamination. But the problem is bigger than that. As long as cheap fillers, such as chondroitin sulfate, are readily available, the risk of contamination exists. Under today's regulatory system, the manufacturers and distributors of drugs are primarily responsible for overseeing the suppliers of active ingredients, but both Baxter International and SPL failed to do so. Baxter International did conduct its own inspection of the plant and later admitted to having found some problems at the Changzhou SPL plant, but it refused to reveal details of the problems to the public. The result was that nothing was done to correct the identified problems, and at least 81 people in the United States died from the contaminated drug.[38]

Cheaper Drugs

Eighty percent of active ingredients in drugs are manufactured in foreign plants and imported into the United States. Still, the pharmaceutical industry and some members of Congress argue that consumers should not be allowed for safety reasons to directly import drugs from Canada and Europe. But prescription drugs are already produced outside the United States with little FDA oversight. The real reason the pharmaceutical industry so fiercely opposes opening up the importation of prescription drugs is that doing so would hurt their profits. Drug prices in Europe and Canada are regulated, and if individuals were allowed to buy drugs from these countries, it would put downward pressure on prices for brand-name drugs sold within the United States.

Without price regulation or competition, Americans are stuck paying excessively high prices for prescription drugs. More than half the respondents in a survey conducted by the Kaiser Family Foundation said they skimped on medical care because of costs. One in five Americans do not fill a prescription for a medicine. And one in six Americans cut pills in half or skips doses, against the advice of their doctors, to stretch their medication longer. There may be some relief in sight. Between 2007 and 2010, more than 100 brand-name drugs with total annual sales of $50 billion will lose their patent protection, opening up the market to the introduction of cheaper generics.[39] With average prices expected to drop by half after the introduction of the second generic, the expiration of patents could translate into billions of dollars in savings to patients and their insurance companies.

But the relief will likely be short-lived. Pharmaceutical companies will try to make up for the competition-induced drop in prices by introducing new, more expensive brand-name drugs. Through promotion campaigns targeting physicians and consumers, pharmaceutical companies try to convince us that their new drugs are better than the old ones. The new drugs may be better, or they may not.[40] The FDA does not require that new drugs be superior to, or even as good as, older generation drugs to be approved. The only requirement is that the drugs be better than placebos.

New drugs may also have unknown side effects that did not show up in clinical trials. One such case is Vioxx. Vioxx was approved in 1999 and quickly became the most prescribed arthritis drug, with annual sales of $2.5 billion.[41] However, subsequent research discovered that Vioxx increased the risk of heart attack by a factor of five, compared to the anti-inflammatory drug naproxen.[42] Five years later, Merck voluntarily withdrew Vioxx from the market. The FDA's own research estimated that the drug caused between 99,000 and 135,000 heart attacks, and resulted in about 28,000 deaths.[43] Sometimes an older drug that has withstood the test of time is the better choice—and the cheaper one.

FIVE

Hospitals

STANDBY SURGERY

I KNEW THAT I WAS HAVING HEALTH PROBLEMS when my name and address showed up on hospital newsletter mailing lists. These lists are sold from one hospital to the next, and soon I was receiving newsletters from almost every hospital in my area. It all started after a minor outpatient surgery in September of 2004. First, Georgetown University Hospital, where I had the procedure, sent me glossy colorful publications with photos of smiling doctors who discussed how to perform surgery. They featured articles on topics such as "Irritable Bowel Syndrome: Getting the Help You Need."[1] Soon, publications from other hospitals followed with articles titled "Outpatient Surgery from Head to Toe," and others on similar topics. Then, invitations to seminars on important topics such as "Legs for Life" and "What If Your Heart Just Stopped?" showed up in my mailbox. One newsletter included a letter from the hospital's president claiming the hospital was "successful and back on track—for good!" which, of course, led me to wonder: were they not on track six months earlier when I had my surgery? My favorite mailing was a letter from Sibley Memorial Hospital asking me "When Did You Last Review Your Will?" It encouraged me to donate money to the hospital when I died.

Clearly, hospitals had tagged me as a sick person with a short life expectancy.

Quality of Care

It is unclear how effective these hospital newsletters advertising surgeries are in convincing people that they need a certain surgery at the hospital being promoted. I didn't put much thought into picking a hospital for the few minor procedures I had. When I had surgery in 2003, my orthopedist had hospital privileges at Sibley Memorial Hospital, so I went there. For the next surgery, I picked Georgetown University Hospital based on the fact that it was a major research hospital. I thought it would be the best hospital in terms of new technology, doctor expertise, and patient services. However, it turned out not to have necessarily been the best choice. According to an article in the *Washington Post* that looked at ratings of Washington area hospitals, Georgetown University Hospital was listed at the very bottom.[2] Based on a list of quality and safety measures, the hospital ranked well below the national average for hospitals in the country.

The federal government and a number of private companies evaluate hospitals based on patient outcomes, quality, and safety measures. The U.S. Department of Health and Human Services (HHS) has developed 27 quality measures of hospital health services (see www.hospitalcompare.hhs.gov). Hospitals are rated on factors such as the percentage of surgery patients receiving preventive antibiotics one hour before surgery, the percentage of heart attack patients receiving a certain drug at arrival, the percentage of pneumonia patients given an initial antibiotic within four hours of arrival, and the percentage of these given the most appropriate ones.

An alternative approach to evaluating hospitals is to look

at health outcomes. The company HealthGrades (www.health grades.com) gives hospitals scorecards based on patient safety and patient recovery results. HealthGrades evaluates survival rates upon admittance, one month later, and again six months later, adjusting for the severity of the disease. Important safety indicators—such as prevention of death in procedures where mortality is usually very low, the absence of foreign body left in during procedure, and avoidance of respiratory failure following surgery—are evaluated and compared to the national average. HealthGrades also provides cost comparisons for certain medical procedures for patients.

Another company, Solucient (www.100tophospitals.com) publishes a list of the country's top 100 hospitals. Evaluation is based on risk-adjusted complications and mortality, patient safety, and average length of stay. Hospitals are also scored on financial outcomes—from the hospitals' perspective—and looks at costs, profitability, and cash-to-debt ratios. If you want surgery at the very best hospital, don't look to the well-known research hospitals. Columbia University Medical Center, Princeton University Medical Center, and Tufts Medical Center did not even make it onto the list.

U.S. News and World Report publishes an annual ranking of hospitals in 16 fields (http://health.usnews.com/health/best-hospitals). A major factor is reputation, determined from a survey of physicians, rather than actual outcomes. A comparison between the *U.S. News and World Report* ranking and scorecards by HealthGrades and Solucient suggest there is little correlation between reputation and performance.

Evaluations of hospitals can provide very useful information for patients. Moreover, hospital scorecards put pressure on hospitals to improve quality and safety measures. In the early 2000s,

Winchester Medical Center in Winchester, Virginia, decided to improve its standing by implementing procedural changes.[3] The hospital reduced the lapse between a heart attack patient's arrival at the door and when treatment was given. It reduced surgical infection rates dramatically by changing the timing for administering antibiotics and by clipping rather than shaving body hair before surgery. By 2007, Winchester Medical Center was ranked highest in safety by HealthGrades and received high marks from HHS.

But what about all the hospitals that did not make it onto the Solucient top 100 list or into *U.S. News and World Report*? What about the hospitals that did not receive an award from Health-Grade or were rated below average by the HHS? Patients still go there for surgery, and by definition, some receive less than optimal care. Some patients, like me, go to substandard hospitals because they do not know better. Some people pick hospitals based on insurance coverage, doctor affiliation, and the commonly held belief that teaching hospitals are bigger and better. Some patients go to a second-rate hospital because it is the only hospital in their community that is covered by insurance.

Surviving a Trip to the Hospital

If you can, stay away from hospitals. The reality is that hospitals are dangerous places. About 240,000 hospital patients die every year from preventable deaths due to human error, bad judgment, or negligence.[4] Every year, five times more people die from preventable deaths in hospitals than in motor vehicle accidents.[5] Hospital-acquired infections especially pose an increasing threat to anyone entering a hospital for medical treatment. Between 5 and 10 percent of hospital patients pick up an infection unrelated to their original medical problems.[6] Viral infections (such as influenza and respiratory viruses) are the most common, but bacterial infections tend to be the most serious and result in more deaths.[7]

Hospital-acquired infections result in about 100,000 deaths every year.[8] The Centers for Disease Control and Prevention (CDC) estimates that treatment of hospital-acquired infections costs nearly $20 billion a year—equal to one percent of the nation's total health care expenditures.[9] Even more worrisome is the increasing number of infections that are becoming resistant to standard treatment. In 1983, the intestinal bacterium, *Enterococcus faecium*, was the first hospital-acquired infection found to be resistant to penicillin. Over the years, the list of drug-resistant infections has grown ever longer.

Fortunately, hospital workers can take preventative measures to limit the spread of infection. Handwashing is one of the most important. In its guidelines on preventing infections in hospitals, the CDC recommends that patients stop their physicians before they touch them and ask, "Have you washed your hands?"[10] Some hospitals have enhanced environmental cleaning, improved communication between hospital staff about patients with infections, and tuck medical charts into plastic pouches. Other hospitals will test patients for infection upon arrival and quarantine them in a special section if they test positive. One Baltimore hospital is asking clergy to wipe down their Bibles so "as to spread only the Word," not the bugs.[11]

Hospital-acquired infections are not the only threat to hospital patients. A patient can fall after surgery and break bones. Busy nurses may not give medication on schedule or may give the wrong medication. Surgical instruments are left inside the body about 4,000 times a year.[12] We have all heard stories about a person who had the wrong leg amputated. This happens about 1,300 times a year. Amputee patients going in for surgery are advised to write "not this one" on the limb they do not want amputated.

A while back, my husband developed an anomalous bump on his forehead. It was not a medical emergency, but over time it started to look rather odd. So he decided to have it removed through simple outpatient surgery. When we showed up for the surgery, an intake nurse informed us that my husband was having a growth on the back of his head removed. My husband corrected her and explained that it was the rather obvious bump on his forehead he wanted removed. Next came a resident doctor who also noted that the growth was on the back of the head. Again my husband corrected her, and she made a note in his patient file that the growth was on the forehead. Over the next 45 minutes, a procession of residents, interns, the anesthesiologist, and anesthesiology interns stopped by, and each one stated that my husband was going to have a growth on the back of his head removed.

Finally the surgeon showed up and took a look at his neck. When my husband pointed out that the growth was on his forehead, the surgeon took out a thick marker and drew large arrows across his face pointing to the bump on the forehead. It worked, and no medical mistakes were made. Despite the fact that my husband told a handful of people that the surgery instructions were wrong, the incorrect information was passed from one person to the next until it reached the surgeon. In this case, the large growth on my husband's forehead was obvious, but still he had a tremendous amount of difficulty correcting the original mistake in his surgical instructions. Imagine the difficulty a very ill patient would have trying to do the same for problems that are far less obvious than a rhinoceros horn on the forehead.

Most hospital-caused illnesses and injuries are preventable. From the hospital's perspective, however, preventing illnesses and injuries costs money. Moreover, hospitals may benefit from hospital-caused illnesses and injuries. After all, patients who fall victim to preventable infections or injuries require additional care, which equals more business for the hospital, often paid for by insurance companies. In the state of Maryland alone, insurance companies paid hospitals an estimated $522 million for treatment of preventable complications in 2008.[13] Extrapolating from Maryland, annual insurance payments on a national level come to $28 billion.

In 2007, Medicare stopped paying for treatment for hospital-acquired infections, falls, and objects left in surgical patients.[14] Soon, other public and private plans followed suit. This move may end up having a considerable impact on hospital practices. Now that hospitals must pick up the tab for treating hospital-acquired infections and other hospital-caused illnesses, they have a strong economic incentive to prevent them from happening in the first place.

Hospitals willing to invest in prevention are able to reduce mistakes. They can do this, most importantly, by ensuring that they have adequate staff. Staffing levels are inversely correlated to medical errors. Overworked medical professionals are more likely to make mistakes.[15] Understaffing of nurses means that they are sometimes forced to work overtime. High patient load and fatigue from long hours can result in inadequate compliance with procedures and less monitoring of patients. Medical residents cited fatigue as a cause for their serious mistakes in four out of ten cases. Overworked hospital staff are more likely to make mistakes because they have less time to talk to the patient to learn about allergies and other information relevant to the patient's situation.

As it turns out, the type of hospital also determines quality of care and patient outcomes. The financial status of a hospital affects the incentive structure, which is reflected in staffing levels, quality of care, incidence of hospital errors, and mortality rates. Hence, the standards of care can vary considerably across public and private hospitals, as well as private not-for-profit hospitals and for-profit hospitals.

The Hospital Business

For-profit hospitals are big businesses. They constitute a rapidly growing share of the industry. Currently, about 20 percent of all private hospitals are for-profit investor-owned hospitals.[16] The largest for-profit hospital corporation is Hospital Corporation of America (HCA). HCA owns 163 hospitals and 105 surgery centers in 20 U.S. states and in England, and it employs 180,000 people. Its annual budget is $30 billion. That is more than 1 percent of total U.S. health-care spending.[17] HCA was founded by the Frist family, which includes Dr. Bill Frist, the former Republican majority Senate leader from Tennessee. While working as a senator, Frist owned a substantial stake in HCA.

In the late 1990s, the U.S. Department of Justice investigated HCA for Medicare and Medicaid fraud. HCA had regularly filed false Medicare reports and had paid doctors kickbacks to refer patients to HCA hospitals. Moreover, it billed Medicare, Medicaid, and the Defense Department's TRICARE for laboratory tests that were not medically necessary; in some cases, the tests were not even ordered by doctors.[18] The investigation further uncovered that HCA routinely engaged in "upcoding," which means that the company assigned false diagnosis codes to patients in order to increase reimbursements from the federal government. Finally, HCA had billed Medicare, Medicaid, and TRICARE for home-health visits for patients who did not qualify to receive them and for visits to qualifying patients that never occurred. The corporation eventually chose to settle and paid the government $1.7 billion, which at the time was the largest fraud settlement in U.S. history.[19]

During his term as senator and majority leader of the Senate, Frist held onto his large stake in HCA. In the Senate, he worked on passing legislation on Medicare prescription drug benefits and setting up health saving accounts; both pieces of legislations would benefit HCA. HCA was also a major source of campaign contributions for Senator Frist. [20]

With uncanny foresight, Senator Frist sold all his shares in the company in 2005. A couple of weeks later, the company's stock plummeted 19 percent in response to a disappointing earnings report.[21] The following year, a Wall Street investment group bought up the company in what was, at the time, the largest leveraged buyout in history.

Supporters of private health care tout for-profit hospitals as both more cost effective and providing better care than not-for-profit hospitals. Research indicates that this is not true. For-profit hospitals are not only more expensive but the care they give is inferior. One study found that hospital costs for Medicare patients were on average 16 percent higher per patient in for-profit hospitals than in not-for-profit hospitals.[22] Despite higher patient costs, patient outcomes are worse. Patients are more likely to die in for-profit hospitals than in other hospitals. One meta-analysis found that the risk of death is 2 percent higher for patients in for-profit hospitals after adjusting for the severity of patients' illnesses and the like.[23] According to the study's authors, this means "14,000 people die each year at for-profit hospitals who would have lived if treated at non-profit hospitals."[24]

One reason behind the higher mortality rates in for-profit

hospitals is that they have fewer highly skilled personnel. Studies have found a clear correlation between the level of skilled personnel and hospital mortality rates.[25] Not-for-profit hospitals generally pay higher wages and are therefore able to attract doctors and nurses with higher qualifications. This translates into better care for patients. Hospital personnel employed by for-profit hospitals are on average paid about 5 percent less (per hour) than private not-for-profit hospital personnel.[26] For full-time registered nurses, the wage differential is even bigger—7 percent. For-profit hospitals have additional expenses, such as paying out dividends to investors who expect a return on their investments, advertising to attract patients, and taxes. Senior administrative officers in for-profit hospitals generally receive higher compensation, including performance bonuses, compared to officers in the private not-for-profit institutions. These additional expenses of for-profit hospitals divert economic resources away from patient care.

Relapse

On the one-year anniversary of my tick bite in Montana, I was feeling better. I was in my second of three rounds of treatment for babesiosis and seemed to be keeping the infection at bay. Hopeful that full recovery was within reach, I took on a job as a consultant doing data analysis of apprenticeship programs. I also started planning for our summer vacation. Because we wanted to spend the vacation with our dogs, and because we didn't have much money as a result of my limited work schedule and expensive medical treatment, we decided on a camping trip in upstate New York. The plan was to take a 30-mile hike through the lake country and sleep in a tent at night. A hiking vacation in tick-infested woods may seem an odd choice of vacation for someone who has spent a year sick with two tick-borne diseases. But I loved the outdoors, and I felt that taking this camping vacation would allow me to face my new "irrational" fear of nature.

Ten weeks before the camping trip, and before I started the third and final round of treatment for babesiosis, my symptoms started creeping back. After I finished this final round, a heavy cloud of fatigue settled over my body. I had a constant headache, and my neck was so stiff I could not bend it forward or to the side. And a brand new symptom presented itself: weight loss. At first I welcomed this new symptom with relief. Ever since I first got sick and became less active, I had been struggling with weight gain, and I was happy that the problem seemed to be remedying itself. But as my weight quickly dropped below my pre-illness weight, I started to worry. I was eating like a lumberjack but was wasting away to nothing. My Lyme disease doctor was not sure what to make of it. He felt that the *Babesia* infection was being sufficiently treated and refused to order follow-up testing. He said that the blood tests would be unreliable because the body can continue to produce antibodies for several months after the infection has cleared. This means that a patient could continue to test falsely positive for Lyme disease and babesiosis even when the treatment has been successful. He speculated that my worsening symptoms were due to a yeast infection from long-term use of antibiotics.

Yeast infections are an unfortunate and potentially serious side effect of antibiotics. Antibiotics kill off not only infection-causing bacteria but also the "good" bacteria that inhabit the stomach and intestinal track to help with absorption of nutrients and keep yeast in check. My doctor prescribed a high dosage of the antifungal medication Diflucan for three days, sold me some herbs to boost my immune system, and recommended a very restrictive diet, low on carbohydrates.

June came along and we went on our summer vacation. The ambitious hiking plans had been scaled back to accommodate my deteriorating health. Instead of a 30-mile hike over six days into the backlands of the Adirondacks, we hiked 3 miles to a lake named Long Lake. It was a beautiful spot with views of the mountains to the west. We set up our tent among the ruins of a grand hotel dating back to the Adirondacks' heyday in the late nineteenth century, when the New York elite escaped the oppressive city heat by retreating to the cool mountains upstate. The hotel closed a hundred years ago; now all that remains is an elegant marble staircase, overgrown with vegetation, leading to the water's edge. It was a magical place—except for the biting insects. We were inundated with black flies during the day and mosquitoes in the evenings. It was also an ideal habitat for ticks: the crumbled hotel walls offered the perfect spot for winter hibernation for animals. There was plenty of blood from a diverse wildlife population to satiate them and low vegetation for questing, which is a term for the way ticks hold onto a blade of grass with their back legs and hold out their front legs, waiting for a passing host. I checked myself for ticks every night but didn't find any. It was still early in the season, and most of the ticks that were active were seed ticks, so tiny that they are hard to spot with a naked eye.

New worrisome symptoms appeared after I returned from vacation, and I don't know whether I was reinfected with Lyme disease while vacationing in New York or I was relapsing. Though I wasn't drinking alcohol, I constantly felt as if I were drunk to the point of being dangerously uncoordinated. I felt dizzy and had the distinct sensation of the ground swaying under me, which made it difficult to walk straight. Blurred vision and slurred speech returned, intensified by pressure building up in my head, as if my brain had become too big to fit into my skull. I stopped driving after

I lost the ability to judge distances and speed. Just being a passenger in a car was nerve-wracking enough, as it constantly appeared as if other cars were about to run red lights and crash into us.

I returned to my Lyme disease doctor with a list of all the new symptoms I had developed since my last appointment with him. He had no explanation for these new symptoms and again refused to repeat my blood tests. He was not concerned that my weight had dropped below 100 pounds; instead, he extolled the benefits of skinniness. I told him that I could barely walk a mile. He told me to try harder. I told him about the bone-breaking pain I had developed in my hip. He told me that an infrared sauna would take care of it.

I was in tears when I left his office. At my first appointment, this Lyme disease specialist had prided himself on his high success rate in treating chronic Lyme disease. He had assured me that I would recover in less than a year under his care. I was starting to suspect that the doctor did not measure his success in terms of test results and clinical presentations of symptoms. Rather, he declared patients recovered as they neared the one-year benchmark. I decided to get a second opinion. I scheduled an appointment with a rheumatologist in the Washington area who had extensive experience in treating Lyme disease. Though my primary problems were of neurological origin, my joint pain, in particular my hips and hands, had become unbearable after I stopped treatment. Sadly, the first available appointment was six weeks out.

That summer of 2004, while waiting for my doctor's appointment, I spent most of the time in front of the computer working on my consulting project. When I had signed on to the project back in February, I had been feeling much better, and the project had seemed like a straightforward task. Now I was struggling to calculate the graduation and dropout rates. I calculated the numbers, found mistakes, recalculated, and each time I arrived at something new. The project leader was getting impatient, and the organization that had commissioned the report was less than impressed with my work. In the end, I asked my husband to finish the report. It was to be my last job; my brain had become too badly impaired by the infection.

Finally, the day of my appointment with the new rheumatologist arrived. She confirmed my worst fears when she told me that I was one of the sickest patients she had ever seen. I protested by saying that I was really not that sick. A physical exam revealed that I suffered from severe peripheral neuropathy caused by damage to the nervous system beyond the brain. The pupils of my eyes were contracting and expanding, causing my vision to grow fuzzy. My response to a tap on the knee with the little hammer was sluggish, and numbness had spread from my toes to my whole foot. She also noted myositis, or inflammation of muscles, and synovitis, a form of arthritis caused by inflammation of the membrane tissue in joints. The test results supported her findings. The tests came back highly positive for Lyme disease, and a polymerase chain reaction (PCR) test found DNA pieces of the *Borrelia burgdorferi* bacterium itself in my blood stream.

Convinced that relapsing Lyme disease was the only plausible explanation for my continued illness, the rheumatologist ordered intravenous treatment with the antibiotic, Rocephin.

The Money Trail

Because of my extensive neurological damage and severe arthritis, my doctor expected the duration of IV treatment to be much longer than three weeks. The rheumatologist suggested that I have a Mediport implanted under the skin in my chest to deliver the medication directly into the bloodstream. This is commonly done

TABLE 5.1 Medical expenses for two minor surgeries,
September 2004 and May 2005

	My medical payments	My health plan's payments	Hospital charges
Surgeon	$ 0	$ 2,382	$ 4,799
Anesthesiologist	0	657	1,206
Device: Mediport	0	878	1,350
Recovery room services	0	617	949
Sterile supply	0	1,119	1,722
Anesthesia	0	161	273
Pharmacy	0	622	1,137
Other services	20	5,507	8,675
TOTAL	20	11,943	20,110

Note: The first surgery was to insert a Mediport for administration of IV antibiotics, and the second surgery was to remove it. The total insurance payment was $8,017 for the first surgery and $3,925 for the second surgery. I paid a copay of $10 for each surgery.

to cancer patients undergoing chemotherapy. The Mediport is inserted only skin-deep, and the surgery takes less than 30 minutes. Normally, local anesthesia is used, but my surgeon insisted that I also receive a tranquilizer so that I would sleep during the whole procedure. This was fine with me, as I had no desire whatsoever to observe what he was doing.

Though the procedures to insert and, eight months later, remove the Mediport, were simple, they were not cheap. The total hospital bill for these two minor outpatient surgeries was an astonishing $20,110. Luckily, my copayment was only $10 for each surgery. My insurance company had negotiated lower reimbursement prices with the hospital and paid "only" $11,943. For example, the total charges for the surgeon came to $4,799, but my plan paid only half of that. The largest billing item was "other services," which were not specified on the explanation of benefits from my health plan or on bills from the hospital. I presume that these are nonspecific charges that help the hospital cover overhead costs (see table 5.1).

The most outrageous charge was $316 for recovery room ser-
vices after the second surgery to remove the IV infusion port.
During that second surgery, every patient's worst nightmare happened to me—I woke up. First I started sensing people in surgery
gowns leaning over me, and then the realization that I was still
on the surgery table hit me. It occurred to me that I should tell
someone, but my still-groggy brain couldn't think of anything
proper to say in this situation. Eventually I mumbled "I think I
am awake." A nice nurse touched my hand and assured me that
the surgeon was just finishing up and that everything was okay.
Fortunately for me, the incision area was locally anesthetized, and
I didn't feel a thing. After the surgeon had sewed me up, I jumped
off the table into a wheelchair. I was taken directly to the dressing
room, had some apple juice, got dressed, and went home. I didn't
spend as much as one second in the recovery room. So, the hospital
basically charged $316 for one small cup of apple juice, of which
my health plan paid $205—a pretty steep price.

With excessive charges for services not even performed, it is
no wonder that national hospital expenditures are growing rapidly. According to data from Centers for Medicare and Medicaid
Services (CMS), national hospital care expenditures increase by
about 7 percent a year.[27] The average hospital cost was $2,567 per
person in 2009. This is an average across the whole population,
including millions of Americans who never set foot in a hospital that year. Hospital-care expenditures are projected to nearly
double over the next decade (see figure 5.1).

Hospital care is the single largest national health expenditure,
accounting for 31 percent of the total.[28] In comparison, physician
care makes up 21 percent and prescription drugs, 10 percent. Some
hospital services, such as heart transplants, are inherently expensive. The surgery itself takes hours and requires the participation

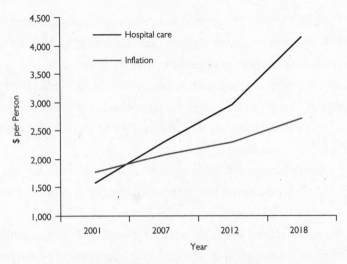

FIGURE 5.1 Actual and projected hospital care
expenditures (per person), 2001–18
Source: CMS 2009: Tables 1, 6.
Note: Inflation is measured by the CPI-W, base 1982–1984=1000.

of a large contingent of hospital staff. The patient spends time
recovering at the hospital after surgery. The development of new
surgical procedures, an aging population, and increasing demand
for expensive procedures all contribute to rising hospital expenditures. Another contributing factor is hospital overhead.

Hospitals have large administrative costs arising from billing and insurance claims. Patients' insurance information has
to be recorded and insurance claims must be submitted. Reimbursements must be recorded and cashed. Patients must be billed
for copayments. If payment is not received promptly, additional
requests for payment must be sent out. Claims denied by insurance will have to be refiled. The administration of insurance
claims and the recovery of payments can be a cumbersome process.
A report by the American Hospital Association found that one

hour of patient care generated 30 to 60 minutes of paperwork.[29] My own experience also suggests that this is the case. From the explanation of benefits statements that my health plan periodically sent to me, I could see that one insurance claim filed by the hospital after my second surgery bounced back and forth between the hospital and the insurance company for seven months before it was finally resolved.

The resulting costs are staggering. A study of acute care hospitals in Florida found that administrative costs accounted for an average of 23 percent of operating costs from 2000 to 2004.[30] On a national level, this translates into about $170 billion in 2009. For-profit hospitals had on average higher administrative costs per admission than did not-for-profit hospitals due to higher salaries and bonuses for administrators at for-profit hospitals and dividends paid out to stockholders.

Not-for-profit hospitals, placed in competitions with for-profit hospitals, act increasingly as for-profit corporations whose main goal is to increase revenues while keeping costs low. Revenues are maximized by charging higher prices for hospital services, providing unnecessary services, and charging for services not even provided. Costs are reduced by cutting staff levels and wages, and postponing the upgrading and replacement of equipment. One rather innovative cost-cutting approach that I encountered during my illness was standby surgery.

Standby Surgery

Yes, there is such a thing as standby surgery. In my case, it was like flying standby around Thanksgiving during a snowstorm, when only a few planes are landing and taking off. In 2004, I needed a minor surgery to correct complications resulting from the infusion device used to administer intravenous medication. A couple of months after having the Mediport inserted under my skin, I noticed a piece of wire was working its way through my skin. I went back to the surgeon, who recommended another surgery to fix the problem. Unfortunately, the surgeon's schedule was booked up for weeks. So his assistant suggested that I sign up for standby surgery. Standby surgery means that you essentially make yourself available for surgery on a given day, and the hospital guarantees that they will fit you in that day—no matter what. This allows the hospital to fit in more surgeries per day without having to set aside the required time for each procedure.

The morning of the surgery I realized it was going to be a long and trying day after reading in the *Washington Post* that Secretary of State Condoleezza Rice was having surgery at the same hospital that same day. I could easily envision the entourage of Secret Service personnel and bomb-sniffing dogs that would follow her into the operating room, while the rest of us patients would have to wait. I never did see Ms. Rice, but my prediction of a long wait turned out to be accurate.

I arrived at the hospital around three in the afternoon and was assured that the surgery would take place soon. After an hour-and-a-half wait, the nurse told me that they were ready to take me down to surgery. Fifteen minutes later, the surgeon came by and told me it was going to be another 30 minutes because the current nurses were leaving at five, and we had to wait for the new crew to come in. It was six before I was wheeled down for surgery. However, they could not find an available operating room, so they placed me in the corner of a dark room. The lighting cast a strange green glow, and the room was freezing cold and smelled of death.

By 6:45, I was still waiting. At this point, I had had nothing to eat and drink since midnight the night before. The long wait, lack of food, and the smell of death were more than I could handle. I broke down, and a nurse rushed to my side, trying to assure me that everything was under control. When that failed, she called for the surgeon. He arrived 15 minutes later with the remains of his dinner still stuck between his teeth. He offered a pill for anxiety, but warned me that if I took it, I would have to wait at least an hour before he could begin surgery. While trying to decide whether to undergo surgery while wide awake or having a panic attack or wait an additional hour, I thought of another solution.

Hours earlier when I checked in, I signed a Patient Rights form. The form stated that at any time and for any reason a patient has the right to refuse surgery. Needless to say, getting off the gurney and walking out would be quite audacious after having already waited for hours. Nonetheless, I got up, took the elevator up to the patient intake room, got dressed, and walked out. For the first time that day, I felt empowered as a patient. The only problem was that I still had the piece of metal sticking out. The next day, I popped a couple of extra-strength Tylenols, pulled my skin away from the Mediport, and with a sterilized set of tweezers, pushed the metal wire back in place. This took care of the problem, and for the next six months until I had the Mediport removed the wire did not reemerge.

Privatization of Hospitals

Before hospitals became a business operated like any other business, there were public hospitals. Public hospitals were established to provide hospital care for people who could not afford to pay for it themselves. They could be found in most American cities. DC General Hospital was the first and only public hospital in Washington DC. It opened in 1806 and provided free hospital services to low-income residents for almost 200 years.[31] DC General Hospital closed in 2001. That same year, the DC government awarded a five-year contract of $375 million to another DC hospital, Greater Southeast Community Hospital, to take over hospital services. At that time, Greater Southeast was a for-profit hospital owned by the Arizona-based Envision Hospital Corporation.[32] Soon thereafter, Envision encountered financial difficulties, and the company filed for bankruptcy the following year.

Envision's financial troubles began following the collapse of National Century Financial Enterprises, an Ohio-based health care financier that offered quick loans to hospitals strapped for cash in exchange for expected future payments from Medicare and Medicaid. National Century would then bundle these loans into collateral for bonds and sell the bonds to investors, charging a transaction fee for the bonds and at the same time passing debt on to investors. But that was not all. National Century was also under investigation by the FBI for making bad loans to Envision and other hospital corporations. National Century had accepted risky collaterals, such as artwork and real estate, in exchange for loans, then passed these loans on to investors, claiming that the loans were backed by secure Medicare and Medicaid payments.

The revelation of National Century's deceptive loan practices set off a cascading effect. When it became known that the loans were supported by questionable collateral, the bundled loan bonds were downgraded, making them less attractive to investors. As investors shied away from National Century bonds, the company soon faced a cash shortage and began to fall apart. Struggling

BOX 5

How to Get Good Care at a Hospital

To get the best care at a hospital, you must be an advocate for yourself as a patient. Enlist family members and friends to be your advocates as well. It is difficult for any patient to both demand proper treatment and avoid being labeled as difficult by hospital staff. Before any medical procedure, many patients will be stressed and overwhelmed and may not be able to think clearly as a result.

A friend or family member can help ensure that you are prescribed the right medications and given proper pain relief, follow-up tests, and procedures in a timely and professional manner. An advocate can also be extremely helpful in communicating any problems and concerns that you, as a patient, might have.

When going in for surgery, patients have certain rights, and also responsibilities, to ensure they get optimal care at the hospital. I wish I had known these things before entering a hospital for surgery:

for-profit hospitals, such as Greater Southeast Community Hospital, were no longer able to obtain loans from National Century, or anywhere else for that matter. The hospital soon ran out of money to pay staff and vendors, and the hospital filed for bankruptcy.

While in bankruptcy, Greater Southeast continued to stay open, but services deteriorated significantly. The *Washington Post* reported "a grim state of conditions."[33] Nurses walked off the job

1. You have the right to decline tests and medical procedures. Even if you agreed to a certain procedure, you can subsequently refuse it for any reason and at any time.

2. Do not assume that information conveyed to a nurse or intern is passed on to the surgeon, even if a note was made in your medical chart. If you have specific medical needs or concerns, you need to inform both the nurses and the treating physicians.

3. Make sure that the surgeon, anesthesiologist, and assisting nurses are in agreement with you about the medical procedure to be performed. If you have any concerns or questions, speak up. In some cases, you might be met with a displeased look and given a hurried answer. If you are not satisfied with an answer you receive, ask again.

4. If you observe a medical mistake, speak up. Many patients observe mistakes while they are being made but do not bring them to the attention of the treating nurse or physician. Do not assume that medical staff knows what they are doing; sometimes they don't.

because they had not been paid. When the hospital failed to pay its suppliers, doctors had to obtain medicines from other medical facilities. Broken equipment was not repaired due to insufficient funds. Patients could not be put on ventilators because the air outlets didn't work. By 2007, the hospital, licensed for 494 beds, operated only 110 beds. Wings of the previously busy hospital now stood empty, while sick patients lined up for care.

The District of Columbia's final solution to the problem was
to sell Greater Southeast Community Hospital to another hospital corporation. The only corporation interested was the New
England–based company Specialty Hospitals of America, LLC.
To sweeten the deal, the city council offered the buyer $79 mil-
lion, including $20 million to mediate purchasing costs.[34] Given
that Greater Southeast was bankrupt at the time and had huge
liabilities, it is questionable whether the hospital was worth anything near $20 million.

The End

The same story has repeated itself across the country as public
hospitals close down, and care is turned over to the private sector. The private sector has failed not only low-income populations without adequate insurance coverage but all Americans.
As illustrated by my own outpatient surgeries, hospital care is
excessively expensive, and the quality of care is less than optimal.
Dividend payments to investors, advertising costs, and an administrative bureaucracy divert resources from patient care. The result
is higher-than-necessary costs that are passed on to Americans
in the form of higher insurance premiums, higher copayments,
and higher deductibles. Wage growth is suppressed as employers
control employee compensation costs in the face of rapidly rising
health care costs. Taxes are higher when taxpayers pick up the tab
for failed private hospitals. All in all, private hospitals, especially
for-profit hospitals, are a bad deal for Americans.

SIX

Laboratories

BLOOD SUCKERS

LIKE LITTLE VAMPIRES, ticks need blood to survive. They lurk in grasses and shrubs, waiting for their next victim, congregating in areas around open water and in transition zones between forests and meadows. Ticks have also taken to suburban backyards, where flowers and other vegetation attract wildlife and provide plenty of opportunity for a meal of fresh blood. The reality is that ticks can be found pretty much everywhere: in all 50 states and even in an urban environment, like Washington DC, with its thriving host population of ground squirrels, garbage-loving rats, and birds.

Without blood, ticks cannot change form from one life-stage to the next, and they cannot reproduce. Many tick species will feed on any mammal, bird, or lizard. The black-legged tick (*Ixodes scapularis*) feeds on at least 125 species of North American vertebrates, including 54 mammals.[1] Its flexibility in terms of food choice has made it one of the most widespread ticks. It can be found in all of the eastern United States and the Midwest. Its cousin, the Western black-legged tick (*I. Pacificus*) is common on the West Coast. Both tick species are culprits behind the transmission of Lyme disease.[2]

Ticks live such surprisingly interesting lives that ours seem mundane in comparison. Their lives can be divided into four life-stages: egg, larva, nymph, and adult. At their larval stage, they are also known as seed ticks and are smaller than the punctuation mark at the end of this sentence. When spring arrives, ticks emerge and climb up a stem of grass, on top of a log, or to the end of a scrub leaf along a path frequented by wildlife, livestock, pets, or people. From this perch they wait for a host. When an animal brushes against the grass or shrub, the ticks grab onto it. Ticks are exceptionally good at locating their unsuspecting hosts because they have sensory organs located on their front legs that detect carbon dioxide, odors, and heat given off by animals.

Once on the host animal, the tick will carefully seek out a site to attach itself. Ticks prefer areas that are moist or hairy, or both—such as ears and skin folds—making them hard to detect. Moreover, tick bites are typically painless, as the tick injects an anesthesia into the bite wound. A tick will feed for several days until it is full. The rear end of the tick is designed to expand multifold as the tick feeds. After a month of digestion, the tick will molt (change shape). Some species can increase up to 600-fold in weight while feeding.[3]

When reaching adult stage, a tick has only one thing on its mind: reproduction. To attract the opposite sex, adult ticks emit sex pheromones. They will often meet up on the host, mate in the host's lush fur, and then eat their last meal. The female dies after laying eggs. The male will mate with several females before perishing.

Ticks harbor hundreds of diseases. Their guts contain viruses, bacteria, and piroplasms. These microorganisms migrate to the tick's saliva and are injected into the host as the tick feeds. The microorganisms normally take hours to reach the saliva, so

frequent tick checks and prompt removal of any ticks are important in preventing tick-borne infections. Recent research has
found that tick saliva also contains bioactive proteins that suppress the host's immune response to tick-borne bacteria.[4] Another
chemical found in the saliva encourages the reproduction of these
infectious germs.[5] This suggests that ticks are not passive transmitters of diseases but actually play an active role in the promotion
of tick-borne diseases in their hosts.

In the United States alone, there are 90 species of ticks, and 15
have been identified as vectors that transmit diseases to humans.[6]
Ticks are most dangerous when they are nymphs, for they are
smaller and harder to detect than adult ticks, plentiful in the summer, and common carriers of diseases.[7] Many tick-borne diseases
cause serious illnesses, some associated with fairly high mortality
rates if undiagnosed and left untreated. Some have chronic stages
with debilitating symptoms that may require lengthy treatment.
Another potentially deadly problem deriving from a tick's bloodthirsty lifestyle is tick paralysis (tick toxicosis). This is not infectious, like Lyme disease. Rather, it is caused by a toxin injected
by the tick while it feeds. Tick paralysis starts in the hands and
feet, then within a week spreads to the face, resulting in slurred
speech and uncontrolled movements of the eyes. The final stage
is paralysis of the heart muscle, which is fatal if not treated. The
cure for tick paralysis is simple: find the tick and remove it. Once
the tick is removed, the symptoms dissolve in the reverse order in
which they appeared, and the patient recovers.

Ticks were not the only blood-loving creatures I encountered
during my illness. Over the years, numerous doctors eager to diagnose me with everything from syphilis to rheumatoid arthritis
have ordered the drawing of countless vials of blood from my veins.

Diagnostic Industry

The importance of diagnostic tests in the detection of illnesses has been growing over the last decade, as physicians increasingly rely on testing for the diagnosis and screening of diseases. Ordering a blood test is quicker than taking a detailed patient history and performing a thorough physical exam. Annual checkups with busy physicians often take less than 10 minutes. The medical diagnostic industry has expanded into a $30 billion industry that employs about 220,000 people.[8] The largest diagnostic laboratory in the country is Quest Diagnostics, which in 2008 had world market sales of $7.2 billion.[9] The New Jersey–based company operates 2,100 patient service centers, 150 rapid response laboratories, and more than 30 regional testing laboratories. The company's 45,000 employees perform more than one million tests each day.

Quest Diagnostics is an American success story. Established in 1996 and driven by venture capital, Quest Diagnostics expanded exponentially by acquiring other diagnostic laboratories, such as American Medical Laboratories in Virginia, and Unilab Co. in California.[10] The purchase of SmithKline Beecham Clinical Laboratories in 1999 made Quest the largest provider of diagnostics testing services in the country. Between 2000 and 2006, market sales increased by 50 percent, from $3.4 billion to $6.3 billion. Over the same period, profits increased by a stunning 250 percent. Quest Diagnostics is a publicly traded company on the New York Stock Exchange (symbol "DGX"), and its success has been reflected in its stock prices, which increased sixfold, from less than $10 per share in 2000 to $64 per share by 2006.

Quest Diagnostic is significantly larger than its main competitor, Laboratory Corporation of America, known as LabCorp, for short. LabCorp employs about 23,500 workers and has annual

TABLE 6.1 Comparison of list price and negotiated prices for selected diagnostic tests, 2005–06

	List price	Negotiated price	Percent difference	Lab	Date
Comprehensive	$64.49	$8.47	661%	QD	5/06
metabolic panel	20.75	3.13	563	LC	8/06
Hepatic (liver)	46.25	6.55	606	QD	5/06
function panel	28.94	2.66	988	LC	6/06
Thyroid stimulating hormone	114.69	13.46	752	QD	5/06
Rheumatoid factor	57.79	4.55	1170	QD	5/06
Lyme disease— Western blot	115.88	12.41	834	QD	11/05

Source: Explanation of benefits statements provided by author's health plan, from November 2005 to August 2006.
Note: "QD" is Quest Diagnostics and "LC" is LabCorp.

revenues of $4.5 billion.[11] Together, the two laboratories have a stronghold on routine testing, serving the majority of physicians, clinics, and hospitals in the United States.

The success of Quest Diagnostics and LabCorp is a direct result of their agreements with health insurance companies. Health insurance companies have negotiated prices with LabCorp and Quest Diagnostics that are substantially lower than those the two labs charge patients directly. For example, Quest Diagnostics' list price for a liver function panel blood test is $46.25; however, my health plan had negotiated a price of only $6.55 for the same test (see table 6.1).[12] This means that my health plan paid only about one-seventh of what I would have paid out of pocket. In return for lower prices, my health plan and other health plans steer patients to these two laboratories through low deductibles and limited coverage of out-of-network laboratories.

The fact that Quest Diagnostics and LabCorp are willing to accept prices that are one-seventh of the list price suggests they have profit margins of over 500 percent on tests paid out-of-pocket. More disturbing is that these excessive markups are primarily paid by people who do not have health insurance coverage, often because they cannot afford insurance. If I had lacked insurance, I would have paid a total of $18,390 for laboratory tests to Quest Diagnostics in 2005.

This huge discrepancy between the list price and the negotiated price gives laboratories a strong financial incentive to bill patients directly at the higher list price, even though the tests are covered by insurance. Quest Diagnostics has repeatedly billed me directly for laboratory tests rather than billing my health plan, in the hope that I would not realize that the tests were covered and would pay prices that averaged six times higher. Legally, a laboratory cannot bill a patient above the copay if the laboratory is in the network of the patient's insurance plan. This means that the laboratory cannot bill patients for tests that the insurance plan refused to pay for. But laboratories regularly do so, hoping patients will pay up.

Lab Testing

The first thing I noticed, as I entered the small windowless room, was the stifling air. Two Hispanic laborers were chatting, a young mother from Africa was quietly talking to her baby, and an old man was mumbling to himself. Some people appeared to have been waiting for a long time, some were even dozing off. We were here for different reasons but were waiting for the same thing. After I stood for five minutes, the pain in my arthritic hip got noticeably worse. I had been keeping an eye out for one of the hard plastic chairs to sit on, but the only chair that became available while I was waiting was quickly claimed by an elderly Indian lady dressed in a colorful sari.

I was feeling sick. But I was probably not as sick as many of the people waiting, if their looks were any indication. Another 10 minutes passed, and I began to contemplate all the exotic and highly contagious diseases people could be harboring. As I envisioned the viruses and bacteria floating in the air in search of a new host—somebody like me with a weakened immune system—I felt sicker. After another five minutes, I couldn't stand it anymore and left to head home for bed. Tomorrow I will make another attempt to have my blood drawn.[13]

At the time I wrote this in my journal, I was 24 months into my treatment for chronic Lyme disease and babesiosis. I had changed doctors twice. I had completed two rounds of intravenous antibiotics and was feeling better. In particular, my brain fog had lifted and my joint pain had eased. But I was far from well. The rheumatologist was a methodical doctor, and she tested me for every conceivable disease that could explain my illness. At one appointment, a total of 18 vials of blood were drawn. The tests for lupus, herpes, thyroid disease, B-12 deficiency, hepatitis, syphilis, Legionnaires' disease, typhus, the parasite trichinella spiralis, and Q-fever came back negative, as did tests for obscure diseases I had never even heard of. The tests for heavy metals and other toxins revealed nothing. Curiously, the test for salmonella, a bacterial infection associated with food poisoning, came back positive for five different strains. As I had no stomach problems, the tests were dismissed. Only the test for babesiosis came back highly positive for the West Coast strain. My months of babesia treatment had utterly failed. I had relapsed and had to start over with treatment.

In November, three months after being tested for almost every conceivable disease, I received a bill for $231.33 from Quest Diagnostics. I had made it a habit to immediately call the billing department to let them know they had made a mistake if, that is,

I was feeling well enough that day. If I was not well enough, my husband called on my behalf. As a result of my slippery memory and physical exhaustion, matters not dealt with immediately soon disappeared into a big black hole.

Sometimes, the customer service representative would tell me that I was billed directly because I do not have insurance coverage. Other times, the service representatives would insist that I had not met my deductible (in spite of the fact that I don't have a deductible). I suspect that service representatives have been trained to offer these explanations to any customer who calls to inquire about billing, regardless of the person's specific health plan. The people who answered the phone also deployed a number of diversionary tactics. For example, they repeatedly claimed that the tests were not covered by my plan and referred me back to my insurance company.

When I called the billing department this time, the person I spoke to agreed to forward the bill to my health plan. The next day, another bill arrived in the mail, this time for $192.67. Thinking the matter had been resolved, I was surprised to receive yet another bill for $74.37 for the same tests a few months later. I called Quest Diagnostics' billing department and was now told that they had submitted the claim to my health plan but had not heard back, so they were billing me instead. This was in February, and the tests were done in August. So I was billed the $74.37 nearly five months after the tests were done. When I called my health plan, the customer service representative expressed surprise that I was being billed, as my insurance company had paid for these tests back in November when I had received the first bill.

When the laboratory sent me a bill for $1,071 in March, we decided we'd had enough. My husband wrote a letter to the laboratory requesting that they stop their fraudulent billing practices.

In the letter, he wrote, "I am writing in reference to a bill that you sent to my wife, Helene Jorgensen . . . I am getting involved because my wife suffers from chronic Lyme disease. That is why she must have frequent tests. Apparently, your lab suffers from serious billing problems." He then noted, "It seems quite clear that you are deliberately billing sick patients, for money they do not owe, in the hope that they will be either sufficiently confused or intimidated enough to make these payments. Let me assure you that in our case, this will not be a way to increase your profits. This is a despicable practice, which also happens to be against the law."

He ended the letter by writing, "I hope that you promptly change your billing practices to comply with the law." The letter worked its magic. One week later, we received a bill for my copay of $10. Over the next many months, I didn't receive a single bill above my copay. Then, a full 15 months after I had had the blood tests done, Quest Diagnostics billed me yet again for $192.67 and $231.33 for the abovementioned tests. My husband called Quest Diagnostics to complain. The service representative acknowledged that this bill should never have been sent to us. She explained that their "computer system periodically kicks out unresolved cases that are then billed to patients."

According to this service representative, the laboratory sends out bills directly to patients themselves for laboratory services for which payments are being disputed by the patients' insurance companies. Though not legal, laboratories get away with it because patients are confused about what they are being billed for and are often too sick to challenge incomprehensible bills. Some patients pay the bills, thinking that they are responsible for outstanding charges. Other patients are simply too sick to deal with bills for tests done many months before, and they choose to ignore them. This can be a dangerous strategy, as the laboratory may eventually turn the patient's unpaid bills over to a collection agency. Such billing practices basically take advantage of the very sick, who will typically have the largest laboratory bills and be the least able to challenge incorrect billing.

False Negatives

Diagnostic testing is, without a doubt, an extremely helpful tool for ensuring timely and accurate diagnosis of disease. But diagnostic testing can have its pitfalls. The doctor, first of all, needs to order the correct test. In my case, the diagnosis of babesiosis was delayed eight months because the doctor had not ordered the right test for it. Second, the test has to be reliable. In order to be reliable, a test must be both sensitive and specific. A sensitive test can accurately detect the presence of an infection; and a specific test can accurately determine that a healthy person is not infected. Often, there is a trade-off between a test's specificity and its sensibility. For instance, a very specific Lyme test avoids misdiagnosing uninfected people with Lyme disease, but it sometimes misses infections in people with Lyme disease.

The example of Lyme disease is particularly useful in evaluating the drawbacks of laboratory testing as a primary diagnostic tool. Both under-testing and unreliable tests stand in the way of diagnosis for many Lyme patients. Physicians outside areas where Lyme disease is highly endemic may not be aware of the presence of Lyme disease, so they do not consider Lyme disease in their differential diagnosis. Moreover, testing is no guarantee of diagnosis. Sometimes the test comes back with a false negative, showing no or low levels of antibodies, even though the patient is highly infected.

This happens more frequently than one would expect. The

ELISA test is the most common one used to detect antibodies against Lyme disease.[14] The test is not a good one; in fact, it is a terrible test for the diagnosis of Lyme disease. The sensitivity of the test is between 40 and 95 percent, which means that the test misses between 5 and 60 percent of cases of Lyme disease.[15] False negatives are more likely to show up in patients who were recently infected and those with late-stage Lyme disease.[16] It can take up to four weeks for the body's immune system to produce a disease-specific antibody response. Patients who are tested too soon may not show a high level of antibodies in response to the disease. Likewise, patients with a chronic infection may not show an immune response, as the Lyme bacteria suppress the immune system.

To make matters worse, studies have found a huge variation in the sensitivity of Lyme tests across laboratories. In one study, the researchers sent 18 blood samples from patients with Lyme disease to five different laboratories in New Jersey.[17] One laboratory detected Lyme bacteria in only 8 of the 18 samples using the ELISA test. The "best" laboratory found 16 out of 18 samples positive. Several laboratories reported inconsistent results. When analyzing split samples from the same patient, they would find one sample positive and a second sample from the same patient negative. Clearly, all laboratories are not the same. In my experience, tests conducted by laboratories that specialize in a narrow range of medical testing are often more reliable than those done by large commercial laboratories that offer a wider range of tests.

Specialized Laboratories

With the growth of Quest Diagnostics and LabCorp through their acquisitions of other laboratories, the diagnostic industry has become highly concentrated. But it has also become more specialized. A growing number of small independent laboratories have been established over the last two decades. These smaller labs are highly specialized, each offering a narrow range of tests for the diagnosis of specific medical conditions. Often the tests offered by a specialized lab were developed and patented by the laboratory's founder, who created the lab to cash in on his or her invention.

A patent gives the laboratory the exclusive right to utilize the test for a twenty-year period. This means that a particular patented test can only be performed by the laboratory that holds the patent. Under the World Trade Organization's (WTO) rules, the patent holder has the right to apply for patents in foreign countries and to be covered under patent protection in those places as well. For example, a laboratory that holds a patent for an HIV test can take out a patent in India, thereby excluding laboratories in India from using the same test for the duration of the patent. If the patent holder then decides not to establish a business in India, Indian HIV patients would be unable to get tested using this particular HIV test. During the term of the patent, the patent holder does not face competition from other laboratories and can therefore charge a higher price for the test. The above-market price allows the patent holder to recover the costs of research that went into the development of the test. If the test is novel with few equivalent alternatives, the monopoly price can be substantial.

In 2006, a naturopathic doctor I had consulted for intense headaches and inflammation recommended tests for allergies. She ordered them to be done at the ELISA/ACT Biotechnologies LLC, a laboratory specializing in allergy testing. ELISA/ACT Biotechnologies offered a comprehensive test that looks for reactions to 200 allergens, including food items, molds, and environmental chemicals. The price tag for the test was $1,260, payable in cash or check only. However, people whose health plans did not cover the tests were given a discount of $660. My health plan covered 64 percent of the cost, leaving me with a bill of $455.

For an additional $200, which for some reason was not covered by insurance, I could be tested for another 20 allergens not included in the comprehensive test. The laboratory offered to send a nurse to my home to draw the blood for $35. Because I was not allowed to eat or shower for 12 hours before the test, and I knew I would be feeling even crappier than usual, I gladly paid the $35, which of course was not covered by my insurance. In total, I spent $690 on the allergy testing. The test results showed reactivity to only six items, four of which I was not exposed to. For my $690, I also received a glossy, bound 15-page report; a laminated card listing my six allergies; a 10-page supplement on exercise, detoxification, and living healthy; and a phone consultation with a nutritionist.

The naturopathic doctor, I later learned after my insurance company refused to reimburse the cost of consultations, was practicing without a medical license.

Two years later, I decided to follow up on the allergy question, and I consulted an allergist. The skin prick test found a severe reaction to dust mites. Dust mites were not included in the ELISA/ACT test, despite it being a fairly common type of allergy. I cleaned up the dust and the mites that thrived on it, and felt better. The allergist was recommended by my health insurance company as she met their "quality and cost efficiency criteria," meaning she was covered by the plan and charged little for her services. The allergy diagnosis, including tests, cost me $10 in copay.

It pays to shop around for cost-effective laboratory tests. Unfortunately, it can be frustratingly difficult to find out what tests cost. Large commercial laboratories will typically list prices on their Web sites or provide them over the phone. But many specialized laboratories do not list prices and refer patients to the ordering physician for pricing information. One reason for the lack of transparency in pricing is "differential pricing," as discussed above.

Other laboratories allow physicians to charge a markup for using the tests. They do so as compensation for ordering the tests and collecting blood samples. The markup between the laboratory's price and the doctor's price is essentially a monetary bonus to the physician to cover administrative costs of drawing the blood, handling it, and shipping it to the laboratory. The more tests a physician orders, the higher the bonus.

The endocrinologist I was seeing for my hyperthyroid problem insisted on billing me directly for Quest Diagnostic tests that were, at the time, covered under my health plan. The doctor's bill that I submitted to the health plan listed only the name of the test, not the laboratory. The endocrinologist was out-of-network, and because the name of the laboratory was not listed on the bill, my health plan treated the tests as out-of-network. I was reimbursed for only 80 percent of the costs. I ended up paying 20 percent of the high list prices instead of my $10 copay. I considered informing my health insurance company that the tests were performed by Quest Diagnostics but worried that I would be stuck paying the difference between the negotiated price and what the endocrinologist charged. So I kept quiet. The next time I had an appointment with this endocrinologist, I requested to be billed directly by the laboratory. The doctor refused this request, and I again ended up paying much more than I should have.

The Patient as a Consumer

Markups and other compensations for tests give physicians an incentive to order extensive blood work. Busy doctors with a waiting room full of patients find it more convenient to order a long list of tests than spend a long time on a clinical examination and the taking of a detailed patient history. Some doctors may fear overlooking something, however unlikely, and they order tests that may not be particulary pertinent to the patient's symptom history, just to be on the safe side. After all, it costs doctors nothing to order unnecessary tests, as patients or their insurance companies are paying.

Although ordering tests saves time, communicating test results can be time consuming, and many doctors fail to forward test results to patients. In a survey of primary care physicians, 83 percent said that they occasionally delay reviewing test results.[18] And in another survey of community-based and academic medical centers, researchers found that physicians failed to report clinically significant test results in one out of every 14 cases.[19]

I often have found that it can be quite a struggle to have results returned from the doctor as well. My former primary care physician, who has a thriving medical practice in part because he accepts any insurance, is often too busy to get back to his patients with results from the many tests he routinely orders. His policy is to contact the patient only if test results are abnormal. But after he failed to contact me about my positive Lyme test when I was first diagnosed in 2003, I always made sure to follow up on any test. Following my annual checkup in 2006, I called to confirm that my test results were normal. I didn't reach the doctor, but he called me back a couple of days later. I could hear that he was shuffling through the stack of papers on his desk to retrieve my file. He finally located it and sounded rather surprised himself as he went over my test results (probably for the first time) and discovered that my thyroid level was extremely high along with my liver count. I was close to having liver failure. He asked me to

come in the first thing in the morning for a follow-up. The doc-
.tor thought I had thyroid cancer and ordered additional testing.
Fortunately, he was wrong. Needless to say, I was a bit annoyed
that he did not get back to me sooner to convey this important
piece of information.

It would be easier and cheaper for patients if they could circumvent the doctor and order tests directly from a laboratory.
Many states, however, have implemented laws that require patients
to obtain a requisition from a doctor for laboratory testing.[20]
This essentially makes physicians the gatekeepers to lab testing.
A patient must pay for a doctor's consultation to get a requisition
for tests. Some doctors even require a second consultation to go
over the patient's test results rather than discuss test results over
the phone at no charge.

To meet the demand for cheaper and faster tests, in certain
states Quest Diagnostics set up direct-to-consumer laboratories
that offered services to individuals without a doctor requisition.[21]
Popular tests included screening for cholesterol, HIV and other
sexually transmitted diseases, and thyroid, liver, and kidney problems.[22] Lyme disease was also high on the list of popular tests. The
laboratory performed the tests and made the results available to
the patient within a couple of days. If test results were out of normal range, QuestDirect would contact customers by phone and
recommend seeing a physician for a follow-up evaluation.

Direct-to-consumer testing is a controversial issue. Many physicians oppose it, arguing that interpretation of diagnostic testing
is complicated and requires years of medical training. For instance,
a false negative test may cause the consumer to not pursue a diagnosis, despite having symptoms; a false positive, on the other hand,
may lead the consumer to pursue further unnecessary medical

procedures. Only a medical professional, they say, is qualified to determine whether additional testing and treatment is necessary.

Proponents of direct-to-customer laboratories argue that self-testing "gives patients more control over their health and may help in the early diagnosis of diseases."[23] Direct-to-customer laboratories make laboratory testing more accessible and cheaper for consumers, thus making it more likely that a person will take the initiative to get tested. Some diseases, like sexually transmitted diseases, may carry a stigma, and people may be reluctant to ask their primary care doctors for a test. Self-testing may help minimize the spread of these diseases. Direct-to-consumer laboratories also offer patients a relatively cheap way to monitor their chronic medical problems, such as high cholesterol, on a regular basis.

Direct-to-customer testing has another advantage: the test results do not appear on the patient's medical record. Some people may want to get tested for a certain disease but fear that a positive result will prevent them from obtaining medical insurance in the future. Most health insurance companies do not provide insurance coverage for pre-existing medical conditions, or they charge exorbitant premiums. Direct-to-customer testing, when done anonymously, offers the opportunity to keep test results off-limits to health insurance companies.[24] For instance, people with catastrophic health coverage may apply for more extensive coverage if they suspect a medical condition based on the test results from a self-test. At that time, the person will not have actually been diagnosed with the medical condition, as only a physician can make a diagnosis. In such cases, self-testing provides consumers with additional information that can help them choose the optimal insurance coverage based on their individual health needs.

Finally, the debate over direct-to-consumer testing speaks to

How to Avoid Getting Stuck with the Bill for Expensive Tests

1. Ask your physician to order tests from a laboratory covered by your health plan.

2. If you have no health insurance, it makes sense to price shop. Quest Diagnostic and LabCorp charge different prices for the same test, and these differences can be large.

3. Your physician may be familiar with or trust the tests from a specific laboratory. If you do not want to spend the money on a specific test, tell your physician that you cannot afford the test. Most physicians do not appreciate having their recommendations questioned by patients, so cost consideration is often the best argument that a patient can bring up. As a patient, you are not required to take the tests your physician recommends. But your physician may refuse treatment to a patient who refuses to take a certain test.

4. If the test is with an in-network laboratory, you are responsible for only the copay. If the laboratory charges you more than the copay for tests covered by your health plan, you should contact the customer service or billing department at the laboratory right away. The laboratory will interpret your failure to contest an incorrect charge as you agreeing to pay the

amount charged and will hold you responsible. If the service representative is not helpful, ask to speak to a supervisor. Supervisors are generally more accommodating.

5. Contact your health plan to notify them of the incorrect charge. If the laboratory gave you a reason for the charge, tell your health plan representative. I have found my health plan to be very helpful in dealing with billing disputes relating to in-network laboratory tests. However, if the laboratory is out-of-network, you are on your own.

6. If you are too sick to contest a bill in a timely manner, ask a friend or family member to help you.

Remember: Any billing dispute with an in-network laboratory is a matter between your health plan and the laboratory. You cannot be made responsible for any outstanding amount that your health plan refuses to pay. Laboratories will try to pass outstanding charges on to the patient. In 2009, LabCorp began requesting credit card info at sign-in. Don't provide this information. Instead, tell them that you "prefer to be billed directly." Otherwise, LabCorp will apply any remaining balance to your credit card. This means that if a mistake is made in processing the insurance claim, you do not only have to contest the claim but also challenge an incorrect charge to your credit card. Don't let them get away with it.

the matter of whether or not patients have the right to know the status of their own bodily fluids. State laws that prohibit diagnostic testing without a doctor's requisition essentially give physicians a monopoly on access to laboratory testing. If a physician refuses to order a certain test, the patient will live in uncertainty about the status of a disease. This is a problem faced by some Lyme patients. The American College of Physicians recommends against testing for Lyme disease unless the patient has a history of tick exposure, displays clinical manifestations consistent with Lyme disease, or both.[25] Their *Guidelines for Laboratory Evaluation in the Diagnosis of Lyme Disease* states that "patients presenting with such symptoms as arthralgia [joint pain], myalgia [muscle pain], headache, fatigue, and palpitations alone, without the objective signs of Lyme disease, have an extremely low probability of Lyme disease and should *not* be referred for laboratory testing" [italics added]. Based on the American College of Physicians' recommendation, many physicians refuse to order a test for Lyme disease, even if the patient lives or has visited an endemic area. This recommendation, in effect, takes away a person's right to know whether she harbors bacteria causing Lyme disease in her own body. Given physician guidelines against testing for Lyme disease, even in endemic areas, it is not a coincidence that the Lyme test was one of the most popular tests ordered from QuestDirect in 2002.

Sense and Sensitivity

Tremendous strides have undoubtedly been made in the development of new and better medical tests, and the benefits of better diagnostics tests are obvious. With better tests, patients are more quickly and more accurately diagnosed. But diagnostic testing is not an exact science. First of all, the physician has to order the right tests. My babesiosis infection went undiagnosed for eight months because the infectious disease doctor ordered the wrong test. Despite the fact that I was bitten by a tick in Montana, he ordered the test for the East Coast strain of the disease. The test came back negative, and I was treated only for Lyme disease at the time. This simple mistake stole five years of my life.

Secondly, tests have to be accurate. Both false positives and false negatives mar Lyme testing. The uncertainty over diagnostic testing for Lyme disease has spawned a divisive disagreement over whether or not to treat patients who test negative for Lyme disease but have clinical manifestations of the disease. This disagreement has fueled one of the greatest controversies in the history of medicine.

SEVEN

Lyme Disease

TWO STANDARDS OF CARE

YEAR 2005 WAS THE ABSOLUTE LOW POINT of my illness. I was undergoing aggressive therapy for babesiosis, but I was not absorbing the medication well, and the infection was becoming drug resistant. Even worse, my Lyme infection blossomed after my doctor shifted the focus of her chemical attack to the babesia blood piroplasms. The joint pain returned along with a long list of neurological symptoms. In particular, my brain was seriously affected by the feasting Lyme bacteria. From an early age, I had been good with numbers, but I became unable to count backward from 100 by subtracting 7: 100, 93 . . . Around 79, I would invariably get lost. Writing was an even bigger struggle. My vocabulary had shrunk to that of a five-year-old. Common words all of a sudden seemed unfamiliar. I knew I was in trouble when I mulled over the spelling of the word "the" and had to look it up in the dictionary to be sure. It was around that time that I started writing this book. My goal was to write at least one paragraph a day. Some days I accomplished only a short sentence before I gave up.

Summer came, and an even bigger problem presented itself. The state's medical board opened an investigation of my rheumatologist, and announced that they would be holding a hearing

to determine whether to formally charge her with medical negligence. This is the first step in revoking a physician's medical
license. I was in disbelief. Here was the most knowledgeable and
professional physician I had ever encountered, who took a detailed
patient history and did a thorough clinical exam at every visit.
Before diagnosing me with relapsed Lyme disease and babesiosis, she had carefully ruled out any other diseases. How could it
happen that this diligent physician, who had successfully treated
thousand of patients with Lyme disease, was facing charges by the
medical board for her treatment of Lyme disease?

It turns out she was not the only Lyme disease specialist being
investigated. An infectious disease physician in North Carolina,
who had published scientific articles about HIV/AIDS and conducted research into the treatment of Lyme disease, was also being
investigated for treating Lyme disease with antibiotics for more
than four weeks. A renowned pediatrician specializing in Lyme
disease was facing charges by the Connecticut medical board
for malfeasance. In the 1990s, dozens of Lyme disease specialists were investigated.[1] Sometimes, the investigations went on for
years without the doctor being formally charged. In other cases,
the charges were dropped after a formal hearing. In a few cases,
doctors were disciplined, often for minor infractions, and placed
on probation. A leading Lyme disease specialist from Long Island,
New York, was disciplined and placed on probation for two years
for his treatment approach.

In early October 2005, I drove 50 miles to Fredericksburg,
Virginia, to attend the medical board's hearing against my doctor.
About 100 other patients and their families had also made the
trip, and the hearing had been moved to a Holiday Inn confer-
ence room to accommodate the huge public interest in the case.
The board's case was based on three complaints from the same

infectious disease physician in Richmond, Virginia. None of the three patients had filed complaints against my doctor. In fact, one patient had refused to release her medical files to the board until she was informed that she could face prison if she did not cooperate with the investigation. The allegations against my doctor were that she had inappropriately diagnosed the three patients with Lyme disease based on a test called the polymerase chain reaction (PCR), a test that detects genetic material (DNA) of the Lyme bacteria, and that she had treated the patients with intravenous antibiotic for more than four weeks.

My doctor came well prepared to the hearing. She detailed the three patients' medical history of Lyme disease; and she described the recovery of the two patients who had followed her treatment recommendations. The third patient had terminated treatment early and was still sick. She presented peer-reviewed research that supported the PCR as an accurate diagnostic test. She explained why the PCR test was preferable to the more commonly used indirect tests, like the ELISA and the Western blot tests. While the PCR test looks for the presence of the *Borrelia burgdorfei* (*Bb*) bacterium in patients with chronic infections, the ELISA and Western Blot tests search only for antibodies against the *Bb* bacterium. During cross-examination, she impressed everybody with her profound knowledge of the research on Lyme disease. The board's expert witness came across as much less impressive. When questioned by the chair of the board about the antibody response to Lyme disease, the expert stated that he was not an expert in Lyme disease and did not know the answer. The otherwise quiet audience let out a discernable gasp. This expert had criticized my doctor's medical expertise, yet he admitted he was not even knowledgeable about the research on Lyme disease.

After the hearing, the board convened behind closed doors

while we patients and our families waited nervously. It took the board less than two hours to come to a decision. The board dropped all charges against my doctor and ended its investigation. The audience broke out in cheers, and some people cried in relief. The state board of medicine had acknowledged that long-term antibiotic treatment of Lyme disease was not medical negligence but a difference in medical opinion.

Lyme Disease

Differences in medical opinion have haunted Lyme patients for years. Lyme disease was first reported in 1909 by a Swedish dermatologist, Arvid Afzelius. A European strain of Lyme disease, *Borrelia afzelii*, would subsequently be named after him. Dr. Afzelius described a case of a woman with a rash, shaped like a bull's-eye, which he called an erythema migrans (EM). Soon, similar rashes were showing up across Europe. In 1922, the connection between the EM rash and ticks was made after a French sheep farmer was bitten by a tick and developed a rash. The farmer soon developed swollen glands, meningitis, and excruciating pain that even morphine failed to dull. After the development of penicillin in 1942, some European doctors began treating patients with antibiotics.

In 1975, Lyme disease was rediscovered in the town of Lyme, Connecticut. A mother noticed that she and her four children came down with rashes, joint inflammation, and pain each spring. Polly Murray later told her story about the discovery of Lyme disease in her book *The Widening Circle*. Talking to other parents in the area, Murray learned that a number of other children suffered from the same medical predicament, and she contacted her state's health department. A young ambitious doctor named Allen Steere, who had just joined the rheumatology department at Yale

University, was sent out to investigate. Dr. Steere recognized that something unusual was going on in the town of Lyme, and he set out to document this apparently unknown disease. Dr. Steere thought that the arthritis was caused by a virus and coined the name "Lyme arthritis" to describe it.

At the same time, William Mast and William Burrows, two doctors with the Naval Submarine Medical Center, also in Connecticut, encountered a handful of patients who had developed a rash and subsequent aches and pains. They successfully treated the patients with antibiotics and hypothesized that Lyme disease was caused by a bacterium. Despite the success of antibiotics, the Yale doctors insisted that a virus was the culprit behind Lyme disease. As antibiotics are ineffective in treating viral infections, they dismissed antibiotic therapy. The debate over the cause of Lyme disease was finally resolved in 1981, when Willy Burgdorfer, an entomologist with the government-run Rocky Mountain Laboratories in Montana, discovered that Lyme disease is, in fact, caused by a spiral-shaped bacterium called a spirochete. The bacterium was named *Borrelia burgdorferi* in his honor. Although Dr. Burgdorfer's discovery settled the debate over the cause of Lyme disease, to this day the debate continues over almost every other aspect of the disease.

The Debate

In 1979, a Harvard entomologist by the name of Andrew Spielman "discovered" that Lyme disease was transmitted by a new deer tick species, *Ixodes dammini*, that could be found only in a small geographic area in New England. By definition, people outside the range of *I. dammini* could not have Lyme disease. However, it soon became apparent to researchers that Lyme disease was not confined to New England. Dr. Burgdorfer detected *B. burgdorferi* bacteria in black-legged ticks (*I. pacificus*) collected in California for his groundbreaking research.[2] As early as 1970, Dr. Rudolph Scrimenti, a dermatologist from Milwaukee, Wisconsin, published an article about a patient with an EM rash who had been successfully treated with antibiotics. Further historical detective work showed that Lyme disease is far from a new disease in the United States. One study detected *B. burgdorferi* DNA in museum specimens of white-footed mice from 1889, suggesting that the disease has been with us for centuries, perhaps longer.[3] In 1992, Dr. James H. Oliver proved that the *I. dammini* tick was not a new tick species; it was the common black-legged tick (*I. scapularis*) found everywhere from Maine to Florida, in the Midwest, and on the West Coast.[4]

The black-legged tick is not the only vector of Lyme disease.[5] How widespread Lyme disease is and how many cases occur each year continue to be subject to debate. The CDC, the federal agency that monitors the spread of diseases, reported 28,921 cases of Lyme disease in 2008.[6] Connecticut, Delaware, and New Hampshire had the highest incidence rates. However, the CDC acknowledges that its strict case definition results in an undercount in the actual number of infections. A report by the CDC notes, "Surveillance of LD [Lyme disease] is subject to several limitations. Studies from the early 1990s suggested that LD cases were underreported by six- to twelve-fold in some areas where LD is endemic; the current degree of underreporting for national data is unknown."[7] The Lyme Disease Association (LDA) estimates that the number of actual Lyme cases is more than 10 times greater than the reported number.[8]

Just as Lyme disease cases are difficult to count, the disease itself is difficult to diagnose. The telltale bull's-eye rash appears in only 60–80 percent of cases, and often it does not resemble anything

like a bull's-eye, making identification difficult for physicians. As
in the case of syphilis, symptoms of Lyme disease are diverse. Some
patients have primarily arthritic manifestations, other patients have
mostly neurological symptoms, and some patients have nonspecific
symptoms such as headaches, fatigue, and pain. Because of this
diversity of symptoms, Lyme disease is easy to mistake for other
diseases. It is sometimes referred to as the "new great imitator."

To make matters worse, Lyme tests are notoriously unreliable.
As I discussed in the previous chapter, the most commonly used
test, the ELISA, misses between 5 and 60 percent of infections.[9]
The ELISA test, like most tests for infections, looks for antibodies against the infection, not for the presence of the bacterium
itself. Antibodies are proteins produced by an infected person's
immune system to detect and fight the invading infections (antigens). However, people with compromised immune systems may
not produce sufficiently high levels of antibodies to test positive.

A diagnosis may be elusive even for patients who test positive
for Lyme disease. Some doctors are reluctant to diagnose Lyme
disease in patients who do not present objective symptoms, such
as a bull's-eye rash or meningitis, even if they test positive. The
reason is that the body may continue to produce antibodies long
after an infection has cleared. As a result, a positive test proves
only prior exposure and not necessarily the presence of an active
infection. Nonspecific symptoms, such as fever, muscle aches, and
headaches, which are so common in the early stage of Lyme disease, are dismissed as the summer flu, growing pains, or old age.

Even more disputed than how to diagnose Lyme disease is how
to treat the disease. One set of infectious disease physicians argues
that one month of antibiotic therapy is sufficient to eradicate
the bacteria. Another set of Lyme disease specialists argues that
the *Bb* bacterium, which causes Lyme disease, is a very complex

bacterium, and longer treatment courses, with two or more anti-biotics in combination, may be needed.[10] The Lyme bacterium has a large number of functioning genes, at least 132.[11] In comparison, *Treponema pallidum*, another spirochete that causes syphilis, has only 22 functioning genes. Moreover, the *Bb* bacterium has the largest number of plasmids of any known bacterium.[12] In layman's terms, plasmids are blobs of DNA molecules that are independent of the bacterium's main DNA. Bacteria with plasmids are very ver-satile and adaptable because they can change their DNA makeup to fit their environment. For example, they tend to become drug resistant. The *Bb* bacterium has been observed to take difference shapes, including a dormant cyst form.[13] Dormancy, immune-suppressant abilities, drug resistance, and other possible mecha-nisms allow the *Bb* bacteria to both evade the infected person's antibodies and survive antibiotic attack.[14]

The Research

The main reason the optimal treatment of Lyme disease contin-ues to be a contested issue more than 30 years after the disease was documented in Lyme, Connecticut, is that little research has been conducted to settle the debate. Most research has focused on comparisons of different types of antibiotic therapy, mostly on patients in the early stages of Lyme disease. Research that looked at patients in late stages of the disease found that the majority of patients recovered following two to four weeks of antibiotic therapy—but some did not. As seem from table 7.1, failure rates range from 10 to 69 percent. Patients with neurological Lyme dis-ease are more likely to fail treatment than patients with arthritis.

The National Institutes of Health (NIH) is the nation's lead-ing disease research institution. It conducts and supports medical

TABLE 7.1 Duration of antibiotic therapy and treatment failure in Lyme patients

Study	Year	Patient group	Therapy	Findings
Lugigian et al.	1999	18 patients with neuropathy	30 days of IV	23% of patients had failed treatment 6 months later. One patient was re-treated.
Treib et al.	1998	44 patients with neuropathy, pain, and headache	10 days of IV	50% of patients continued to report cognitive problems and fatigue 3–5 years after therapy. Patients continued to test positive for Lyme disease.
Oksi et al.	1998	60 patients with neurological and musculoskeletal symptoms	100 days of oral or 14 days of IV + 100 days of oral	10% failed treatment or made only moderate progress.
Wahlberg et al.	1994	92 patients with late-stage Lyme disease	14 days of IV, or 14 days of IV + 100 days of oral	69% failed the 14 days of therapy, and only 13% failed 114 days of therapy.
Lugigian et al.	1990	27 patients with encephalopathy	2 weeks of IV	22% of patients relapsed after 6 months; 15% never improved
Dattwyler et al.	1988	23 European patients with late-stage Lyme disease	2 weeks of IV	26% failed treatment

research on disease prevention and new treatments. The NIH grew from a one-room laboratory studying cholera and other deadly diseases brought to the country by seamen in the 1880s to an agency employing 18,000 people. The NIH gives out $28 billion every year to fund research. Most of the money (83 percent) is awarded as research grants to universities, medical schools, and other research institutions. The NIH also has its own in-house research staff, which mostly focuses on researching deadly tropical diseases and other health problems with little potential for private profit.

Despite the fact that Lyme disease is the fastest growing infectious disease, and that more than 28,000 new cases are reported every year, the NIH has funded only three studies into treatment for patients who fail antibiotic therapy. These three studies returned mixed results. One, conducted by the New England Medical Center in Boston, examined whether people with a history of Lyme disease and prior antibiotic treatment would benefit from additional antibiotic treatment. Of the 64 patients who received one month of IV antibiotics, followed by two months of oral antibiotic therapy, 40 percent felt better three months after their therapy ended. But about one-third of the patients felt worse. Moreover, the patients did not fare significantly better than the placebo group, of which 36 percent had improved health status. Thus, the authors concluded that "treatment with intravenous and oral antibiotics for 90 days did not improve symptoms more than placebo (see table 7.2)."[15]

Another NIH-funded study conducted by researchers with Columbia University Medical Center found that 23 patients with cognitive impairment caused by encephalitis (brain inflammation) who received 10 weeks of IV antibiotics saw huge improvements in cognitive function, pain, and fatigue (compared to the placebo

TABLE 7.2 Benefits of additional antibiotic therapy in
chronically ill patients for whom prior treatment failed

Study	Year	Patient treatment group	Therapy	Findings
Klempner et al. New England Medical Center	2001	64 patients with neurologic and/or arthritic symptoms	30 days IV + 60 days oral	No difference between treatment and placebo group
Fallon et al. Columbia University	2008	23 patients with encephalitis	10 week IV	Short-term benefits
Krupp et al. Stony Brook University	2003	28 patients with chronic fatigue	4 weeks IV	69% improved

group).[16] However, the benefits were short-lived, and 14 weeks after ending treatment most patients had relapsed.

Finally, a study by researchers with Stony Brook University on Long Island, New York, looked at Lyme disease patients who suffered from persistent severe fatigue despite having received prior treatment.[17] The study found that one month of antibiotic therapy significantly reduced fatigue in the 28 patients in the treatment group. Fully 64 percent of the patients who received the antibiotics, versus 19 percent of patients in the placebo group, showed improvement in fatigue five months after completing one month of therapy.

One reason the studies are inconclusive is that each looked at different patient groups: patients with chronic fatigue, patients with cognitive impairment, and patients with a potpourri of symptoms. Before enrolling in the studies, many of the patients had been sick for a long time. Lyme patients in the New England Medical Center had been sick at least 6 months and some had been sick almost 12 years prior to the study. Patients in the Columbia University study had been sick on average for 9 years, and some patients much longer. Most of the patients had received extensive prior antibiotic therapy for Lyme disease: on average 7.2 weeks in the Stony Brook study, 8.3 weeks in the New England study, and 41 weeks in the Columbia study.

Because the studies enrolled patients who had been sick for a long time and had already received months of antibiotic therapy, they were designed to select patients who had already failed the treatment. Therefore, it is not surprising that most of these hard-to-treat patients did not recover after one to three months of additional treatment. Imagine a cancer study that enrolls women with breast cancer who have failed several rounds of chemotherapy to evaluate the benefits of one additional infusion. By its design, such a study would find that only a small percentage would be cured of breast cancer. If the researchers concluded that additional chemotherapy of any duration was ineffective based on this finding, their study would be dismissed. And if the researchers concluded, based on their ill-designed study, that chemotherapy in general is useless against breast cancer after one initial round of chemotherapy, they would be laughed out of town.

Unfortunately, this is not the case with Lyme disease. The findings of the New England Medical Center's study were published in the *New England Journal of Medicine*, one of the country's most prestigious medical journals.

Two Standards of Care

Due to the split in medical opinion over the diagnosis and treatment of Lyme disease, two standards of care have been developed and exist side-by-side. One standard, based on the Infectious Diseases Society of America's (IDSA) guidelines, recommends two to four weeks of antibiotic therapy and recommends against more than four weeks of treatment. The guidelines state that "antibiotic therapy has not proven to be useful and is not recommended for patients with chronic (more than six months) subjective symptoms after recommended treatment regiments for Lyme disease."[18] The guidelines provide no guidance on further therapy for patients with objective symptoms. Patients who still have symptoms following standard treatment are classified as having "post–Lyme disease syndrome," an elusive diagnosis for which no treatment is known. According to the IDSA guidelines themselves, "There is no well-accepted definition of post–Lyme disease syndrome" for which "therapeutic modalities [are] not recommended."[19]

The International Lyme and Associated Diseases Society (ILADS), on the other hand, argues that many patients who continue to be symptomatic or relapse following initial therapy have a persistent Lyme infection. The ILADS guidelines recommend re-treatment of such patients. Persisting and relapsing infections are believed to be treatment resistant; therefore, combination antibiotic therapy of longer duration is recommended.[20]

Reading the two sets of guidelines representing two different views of Lyme disease is like reading about two completely different diseases. The IDSA guidelines describe Lyme disease as a mostly mild infection, most commonly expressed by a rash that is easily treated. Late-stage Lyme disease with arthritic and neurological involvement is rare. On the other hand, the ILADS guidelines depict chronic Lyme disease as a debilitating disease with severe nervous system involvement that is hard to treat successfully. Cognitive impairment, pain, and neuropsychiatric manifestations are commonly observed in patients with chronic Lyme disease.

Following the IDSA's release of its updated guidelines in 2006, the Connecticut attorney general opened an investigation into the IDSA, charging anti-trust violations. The attorney general determined that the guidelines had been developed based on research that supported short-term antibiotic treatment and dismissed research that contradicted their recommendations. Not a single researcher with alternative views was appointed to the panel that developed the treatment guidelines.

The investigation uncovered "serious flaws in the Infectious Diseases Society of America's (IDSA) process for writing its 2006 Lyme disease guidelines."[21] The chairman of the panel had hand-picked likeminded panelists and had failed to conduct a conflict of interest review prior to appointing them. The investigation further found that the authors of the guidelines had various undisclosed conflicts of interest. Some authors consulted with insurance companies to set standards for insurance coverage of the treatment of Lyme disease. Some consulted with pharmaceutical companies that developed medications to treat chronic arthritis and neuropathy. Nine authors have direct commercial interest in Lyme vaccines. Four of the authors had received research funding to develop diagnostic test kits.

In May of 2008, the IDSA settled with the attorney general, agreeing to create a review panel of independent researchers to review and revise the guidelines. The new panel was required to conduct an open scientific hearing. The settlement sent shockwaves through the medical community. Medical guidelines have been seen as the gold standard for medical treatment, developed by the best medical minds and based on the best available science. But as the attorney general's investigation exposed, the process of developing guidelines can be corrupted when a few experts let their own beliefs and financial interests overrule science. Whether the writing of the IDSA guidelines was an isolated case or the integrity of medical guidelines in general is being eroded by conflicts of interest remains to be seen.

Going to Valhalla

The issue of treatment guidelines may seem like an academic debate among researchers, but it most assuredly is not. Treatment guidelines affect patients directly in terms of treatment options as well as insurance coverage. Based on guidelines developed by medical societies such as the IDSA, health insurance companies set rules on the type and duration of treatment covered. Treatments that fall outside the established guidelines are considered "experimental" and are not typically covered by insurance. In the case of Lyme disease, many patients have found that after four weeks of therapy their health insurance companies refuse to pay for further treatment, even if they are still sick and continued treatment is prescribed by their physician.

Health insurance companies have a direct financial stake in treatment guidelines. The stricter the guidelines, the more health care plans can shift treatment costs onto patients by deeming the treatments "experimental." The Connecticut attorney general uncovered that health insurance companies were paying the panel members who were writing the treatment guidelines for Lyme disease—clearly a conflict of interest.

The IDSA and insurance companies are putting pressure on physicians to treat according to guidelines, even if a patient's case falls outside their bounds. Such pressure is frightening and has tangible ramifications on the decisions physicians make. For example, some physicians will refuse to schedule follow-up appointments after four weeks of treatment, like the infectious disease doctor at the prestigious research hospital I had consulted after my tick bite in Montana. Other physicians will declare their patient cured and write off persistent symptoms to ambiguous conditions such as "post–Lyme disease syndrome," fibermyalgia,

or chronic fatigue syndrome, essentially dooming them to a life
of illness.

Fed up with denial of treatment beyond the IDSA-recommended
two to four weeks of antibiotics, hundreds of people from all parts
of the country gathered in Valhalla on a cold dreary November
day to protest the newly released updated treatment guidelines
by the IDSA.[22] Valhalla, located in New York's Hudson Valley,
is the home of the Westchester Medical Center, the workplace
of Dr. Gary Wormser, the lead author of the IDSA guidelines.
Lyme patients and their families were waving signs reading "DR.
WORMSER—You Make Me Sick"; "Gross Medical Neglect";
and "STOP the Ignorance," referring to the guidelines' recommendation against prolonged antibiotic therapy.

Pat Smith, president of the Lyme Disease Association, gave
a passionate speech at the rally in which she noted, "I cannot
fathom why patients are being subjected to guidelines which say
their disease does not exist, which say treatment is not recommended for them, and which say clinical discretion should be in
effect removed from their treating doctors."[23] Such guidelines are
hard to fathom, especially when you consider that the IDSA recommendations against additional antibiotic therapy for patients
with persistent or relapsing symptoms are based on one faulty
study that found no positive effect from additional antibiotic
treatment.[24] The lead author of this study, Dr. Klempner, is also
an author of the IDSA guidelines, whose lead author is Dr. Wormser, who is the colleague of Dr. Raymond Dattwyler, who is also a
coauthor of the IDSA guidelines and fatigue study. Dr. Klempner
is also an editor of the *New England Journal of Medicine* (*NEJM*),
the journal that published his ill-designed study on additional
treatment. Ever since Dr. Klempner has served as an editor, the

NEJM has not published any articles on persistent Lyme disease that contradict the IDSA's recommendations. Readers will have to turn to other journals to learn about the benefits of prolonged antibiotic therapy, such as studies that have found that *Bb* bacteria can survive antibiotic therapy in beagles, mice, and humans. In a cruel experiment, Cornell University researchers placed Lyme-infected ticks on sixteen young beagle puppies. After three months of infection, the puppies were treated with one month of antibiotics, except for a handful of unlucky puppies who ended up in the control group receiving no antibiotics. At the end of the study, all the puppies were killed. When researchers biopsied the various body tissues, they found Lyme bacteria in all the dogs, those treated and those not treated with antibiotics. They concluded that the bacterium "disseminates through tissues by migration following tick inoculation, produces episodes of acute arthritis and establishes persistent infection. The spirochete survives antibiotic treatment and disease can be reactivated in immunosuppressed animals."[25]

Likewise, researchers at the University of California found that the Lyme bacteria could survive high-dosage antibiotic therapy in mice with chronic infections.[26] Ticks that fed on the post-treated mice became vectors of Lyme disease and infected other mice who were otherwise healthy. Clearly, Lyme bacteria can survive in dogs and mice treated with antibiotics. Why, then, are some doctors so quick to dismiss the idea that the same is the case with humans?[27] I know for a fact that Lyme bacteria can survive three weeks of IV therapy, reproduce, and cause a full relapse in infection. I also know for a fact that Lyme bacteria can be very treatment resistant.

Shortly before Christmas of 2005, my wonderful doctor gave up on me. She told me that I was one of her sickest patients and

BOX 7

How to Prevent Lyme Disease and Other Tick-Borne Diseases

There is currently no vaccine available against Lyme disease. Therefore, it is important to be vigilant when outside. There are five simple steps one can take to lower the risk of Lyme disease:

1. Wear light-colored clothes outside to better spot the ticks before they attach themselves. Ignore the geek factor and tuck pants legs into socks.

2. Spray shoes, pants, and exposed skin with insect repellent with 20–30 percent DEET or permethrin. Put clothes in the dryer for 45 minutes at the high-heat setting upon returning home.

3. It is a misconception that ticks are primarily found in forests. Ticks actually prefer suburban landscaping. Avoid scrubs and tall grass, especially in the spring and early summer when the risk of tick bite is highest. Fordham University in New York puts out a tick index that estimates the risk of ticks in any given week: www.fordham.edu/tick.

4. Around the home, remove leaf litter and clear tall grasses and brushes. Mow the lawn frequently.

5. Do a tick check when returning home and the next morning in the shower. Remember that ticks can be as tiny as a ".."; and look with special care in moist areas, such as behind the knee, armpits, and other skin folds. To get in the mood for a tick check listen to country singer Brad Paisley's song "Ticks."

that I was not getting better. My treatment had turned into a game of whack-a-mole: you treat one infection and the other infection flares up. She was out of ideas about how to get me well. She recommended that I find another Lyme disease specialist who would take a fresh look at my case. Up until this point I had held onto the belief that in another six months I would be better. Rather than saying I was sick with Lyme disease, I would make a point of saying, "I am recovering from Lyme disease"—even if the recovery was painfully slow. For the first time, I feared that I would never recover. The thought was unbearable.

EIGHT

Health Care Reform

RECOVERY

BY THE END OF 2005, my own medical costs had accumulated to $74,000. And along with mounting bills came mounting woes. The first doctor had declared me cured. The second doctor had blamed my continued illness on my "unwillingness to get well." The third doctor had given up on me. For the fourth time I was looking for a new doctor. Rather than staying locally, I decided to seek the medical opinion of one of the leading Lyme disease specialists in the country, who also had experience in treating my obscure strain of babesiosis. The doctor was located across the country, and at the time I made my appointment, I wasn't even sure I would be well enough make the trip.

My husband took time off from work to accompany me to my appointment. At this point, I was too sick to keep track of my own illness and needed his help with everything. When the new doctor asked me about my symptoms, I struggled to remember a single one. Not even loss of memory came to mind. He spent almost two hours with us and concurred with my other doctors that I was very sick, but he was not sure what the underlying problem was and ordered a long list of expensive tests. He didn't make any promises that he would cure me. Still, his extensive knowledge and deep compassion made me hopeful that he could.

Again the tests for Lyme disease and babesiosis came back highly positive, confirming that prior treatment had, indeed, failed. A test for a specific kind of natural killer cells (type of white blood cells) came back abnormally low. A test for inflammation came back abnormally high—15 times the upper limit of normal range. An echocardiogram showed damage to two of the heart valves. I was surprised to find out that the test for cat scratch disease also came back positive, since I have little contact with cats. It turns out that cat scratch disease (*Bartonella henselae*) is named after the scratch-like rashes that infected people develop, not the transmission mechanism. Though a bite from an infected cat can make a person sick, another source is a bite from a tick. My scratch-like rashes had appeared above my right knee the previous summer.

The new doctor treated the *Bartonella* infection, then turned his attention to babesiosis. He prescribed the standard treatment of Mepron. I felt better while taking the treatment, but as soon as it ended, I relapsed. He then devised a clever treatment plan. He would treat with the malaria drug Lariam for three months, then shift to the *Babesia* drug Malarone for three months, then shift to Flagyl, an antibiotic with antiparasitic properties for three months, each in combination with an antibiotic for Lyme disease. He warned me that the treatment was going to be lengthy, given the severity and duration of my illness. The side effects of the medication would make me sicker before I got better. If I was not cured after nine months, he told me, we would start over again—and again—until the infections were under control.

My progress was almost indiscernible, but eventually I began to notice tiny improvements: I found myself lost less often when leaving my neighborhood. I started combining a trip to the pharmacy with a stop at the convenience store before I got exhausted. My afternoon naps became shorter. The walks with my dogs became a little longer. I gained weight. My vision was less blurred and reading became easier. I went to the movies for the first time in years. Instead of struggling for hours over a sentence, I could write two sentences and then a paragraph in a day. I started making plans for the future.

The Economics of Health Care

When I told my Lyme disease doctor that I was writing a book about health care, he asked me to put him in my book. When he had signed up for family coverage with a high-deductible plan, premiums were $140, and he was happy with the plan. But it didn't stay that way. His premium increased 10-fold in about half as many years, and he began paying over a thousand dollars in premiums per month, while coverage diminished.

Soon health care will become so expensive that even doctors will not be able to afford good health care for their own families. To understand how it has come to this, we have to look at the economics behind our health care system. As opposed to the health care systems in other industrialized countries, health care in the United States is primarily a private system that relies on market forces for the allocation of health care services. Economic wisdom states that for standard goods and services, market forces will result in an efficient allocation of resources. But the market for health care is quite unlike the market for standard goods and services.

Take televisions, for example. When buying a new television, the consumer has a wide selection of television manufacturers, types, and sizes to choose from, which can be purchased from a number of different retailers. The characteristics of a television set—screen size, aspect and contrast ratios, display type, and resolution—are printed on the box. Most retail stores have sample televisions plugged in so consumers can judge the picture quality for themselves and get a sense of how to operate them. Though some stores may have a greater selection than others, televisions sold by one store are pretty much the same as televisions sold by another store, making price comparison fairly simple.

In contrast, comparing costs for health care services is next to impossible. Hospitals do not list prices of medical procedures on their Web sites, nor can you just call the hospital and ask. Health care services, unlike televisions, are not uniform. Each person needs specific care based on the individual's medical history. Doctors perform these services differently and may use different technology. Unlike television dealers, who have a selection of TVs plugged in for customers to view, surgeons rarely let you watch a surgery before you sign on to get one of the same. Worst of all, the purchase of medical services is final. If you are unhappy with your medical service, you cannot just return it and get your money back. Reversing a medical procedure is complicated, expensive, and potentially life-threatening.

However, the biggest difference between standard consumer goods or services and medical services is that the former are optional. People can live perfectly happy lives without a 50-inch plasma HDTV. On the other hand, most medical services (except for elective procedures) are medically necessary. A person with coronary heart disease may die without quadruple bypass surgery. People with gallstones need surgery to have them removed, or they will experience a diminished quality of life. People are willing to pay any price for a necessary surgery.

According to economic theory, a good or service must be uniform for the market to provide efficient outcomes; the sellers and buyers must have full information about the good or service, including its price and market conditions; and there must be many buyers and sellers with free entry to and exit from the market. In the case of health care, none of these principles are met. Health care services vary from patient to patient, and the consumers—that is, the patients—typically have limited knowledge of what they are buying. They have even less understanding of the market conditions with convoluted pricing practices. Physicians must be licensed to provide health care, which is good, but it means that the number of providers is limited. Finally, patients cannot "exit" without negative consequences, which in the worst-case scenario is death.

Medical Waste

Because health care is not like standard consumer goods and services, a private health care system relying on market forces is *ineffective, inefficient,* and *expensive.* By placing so many restrictions on health care, a private health care system is ineffective in providing adequate health coverage. The allocation of resources is inefficient, leading to overtreatment of some people with good health coverage and undertreatment of people with limited or no health coverage. The result is a huge amount of waste and the creation of a vast bureaucracy needed to track costs, bill patients, and collect payments.

Administrative costs in the U.S. health care system are enormous. Private for-profit insurance plans take out 10 to 25 percent of premiums for administrative costs before paying out a single dollar for health care services.[1] Meanwhile Medicare keeps administrative costs to less than 3 percent of expenditures. If administrative costs of private health insurance plans could be reduced to the level of Medicare, Americans would save $120 billion per year on health care, enough to provide comprehensive coverage to all the uninsured in the United States.[2]

But Medicare is not available to most Americans under the age of 65. Instead, we have to obtain insurance either directly or through our employers from private insurance companies such as UnitedHealth Group, Aetna Inc., and WellPoint Inc. (the parent company of many state Blue Cross Blue Shield organizations) which are large for-profit corporations, just like Exxon Mobile, CitiGroup, and General Motors.

The largest health insurer in the country is UnitedHealth Group, ranked 25 on 2008's Fortune 500 list of largest corporations. The company was established in 1977 and has since grown at an exponential rate by buying up other health insurance companies across the country. Today, UnitedHealth employs 70,000 people and provides health coverage to over 60 million individuals. Its profits topped at $4.7 billion in 2007.[3] When United-Health acquired PacifiCare Health Systems for $9.2 billion, it held such a large share of the health insurance markets in Arizona and Colorado that it violated antitrust laws and was forced to spin off some of its insurance business.

The success of UnitedHealth did not, however, translate into better health coverage for subscribers. After UnitedHealth bought up my insurance company, I saw my benefits shrink and insurance premiums steadily go up every year. Along with premiums, the company's stocks increased from less than $4 per share when CEO William W. McGuire took over the reins of the company in 1992 to a peak of $64.61 by December 2005. Sorry to say, I did not invest in UnitedHealth. One person who did, however, was the CEO. McGuire's compensation package included a large number of stock options, which gave him the right to buy or sell stocks in the company at a specified price and specified date. So, as the value of UnitedHealth's stocks increased, so did McGuire's compensation.

By the end of 2005, McGuire had $1.6 billion in exercisable stock options.[4] But the stock party came to an end when the *Wall Street Journal* published a series of articles in March 2006 that described how McGuire and other executives had inflated the value of their stock options by backdating them.[5] The backdated stocks were priced as if they were issued at an earlier date when the price was lower. In McGuire's case, his stock options were "issued" over a 12-year period at the absolutely lowest prices, something that is statistically improbable unless he backdated his stock options. Though this is not necessarily illegal, companies that backdate stocks are required to report the practice to stockholders and the Internal Revenue Service (IRS). According to the *Wall Street Journal*, McGuire and other executives had failed to do so.

McGuire resigned under pressure from investigations by the federal Security and Exchange Commission (SEC), the IRS, and the U.S. Department of Justice, though not before the board of directors had approved a severance and retirement package worth over $1 billion, plus lifetime health care coverage.[6] It was one of the largest golden parachutes in the history of corporate America. To put the numbers in perspective, consider this: private insurance companies' health expenditures were on average $2,431 per person in 2006, which means that McGuire's exit package could have paid for almost half a million uninsured people's health expenses for a full year.

Eventually McGuire settled with the SEC. Without admitting or denying any wrongdoing, he agreed to pay back $468 million dollars to his former employer, plus pay a meager $7 million in civil penalties.[7]

The fundamental problem with a market-based health care system is that money underlies incentive structures and allocation of medical services, and CEOs are not the only ones scamming the system. Health care providers try to increase revenues while reducing expenses. Revenues can be increased by raising prices, increasing patient volume (by spending less time with each patient), and overbilling. Some physicians bill for more minutes than they actually spent on the patient's case. Doctors often submitted claims to be reimbursed for 40 minutes when they spent much less time with me. One cardiologist saw me for less than 15 minutes and showed no evidence of having familiarized himself with my case before entering the exam room, yet he still billed for the longer consultation. He would have spent even less time with me were it not for the questions I asked him as he already had one foot out the door. An endocrinologist I consulted billed in-network laboratory tests as out-of-network at a much higher price so he could earn a markup. Another doctor I consulted billed consultations with her nurse as a consultation with a physician, and thus got reimbursed at a higher rate.

Some doctors recommend medically unnecessary procedures to increase business volume and boost returns on their investments in a medical device company or physician-owned hospitals. Not only is this costly but it can also put patients at risk. For instance, MRI and CT scans expose patients to 100-fold the radiation of an X-ray and should therefore be used sparingly. Nonetheless, some physicians who have invested in expensive scanning equipment readily order scans as a first option. Surgeries are fraught with risks, from hospital-acquired infections to complications from surgery to death; still, specialists across the country readily recommend surgery even when nonsurgical alternatives, such as counseling for lifestyle changes, physical therapy, and alternative medicines, are available.

In-network diagnostic laboratories bill patients directly at higher list prices rather than submit the bill to the patient's health plans with which it has negotiated lower prices. Pharmaceutical companies misrepresent the benefits of their new and more expensive drugs in research published in medical journals, in sales pitches to physicians, and in advertisements to consumers. The National Health Care Anti-Fraud Association estimates health care fraud accounts for at least 3 percent of all health care spending, equal to $68 billion annually.[8] The FBI puts the cost of fraud as high as $226 billion.[9]

Waste and fraud translate into higher health care costs for patients and their health insurance companies. Insurance companies seek to reduce their share of costs by denying coverage for expensive care and rescinding coverage for subscribers with high bills. PacifiCare (owned by UnitedHealth Group) was investigated for improperly denying 30 percent of all claims.[10] Blue Shield of California (owned by WellPoint) was investigated for rescinding coverage for minor omissions on the application.[11] Some insurance companies use innovative tactics to discourage people from seeking medical care. In 2002, Kaiser Permanente admitted to paying their telephone clerks in northern California bonuses for reducing the number of doctor visits they scheduled.[12] Clerks that scheduled appointments for less than 35 percent of people who called and kept the conversations shorter than 3 minutes and 45 seconds on average received a bonus.

As a result of high administrative costs, waste, and fraud, health care costs in the United States have been growing considerably faster than in European countries and Canada. According to data from the OECD (Organisation for Economic Co-operation and Development), per capita health care expenditures increased 6.5 percent in the United States between 1987 and 2007, but only

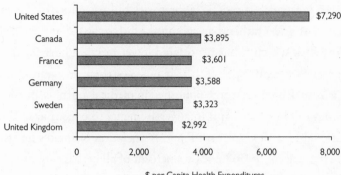

FIGURE 8.1 Per capita health expenditures in selected OECD countries, 2007

Source: OECD 2009.
Note: Amounts are measured in US$ PPP.

4.3 percent in Germany, 5.5 percent in France, and 5.2 percent in Canada. As a result, the gap in health care costs between the United States and these other countries has increased. Americans now spend more than twice as much on health care, on a per person basis, than citizens of France, Germany, the Netherlands, Sweden, the United Kingdom, and Japan. We also spent nearly twice as much as Canadians, $7,290 versus $3,895 per person according to OECD data (see figure 8.1).

Not only is the U.S. health care system more expensive but it fails to produce better health outcomes. Every single western European country has higher life expectancies than the United States.[13] The United States also ranked near the bottom in terms of "healthy life expectancy at age 60," meaning that substantially more Americans spend more of their lives in poor health than do adults in other countries.[14] Even worse, out of 19 countries studied, the United States ranked at the bottom in preventable mortality resulting from bacterial infections, screenable cancers, diabetes, heart disease, stroke, and complications from common surgical procedures.[15] If the United States were to match the number of preventable deaths in France, more than 100,000 lives could be saved every year.

Health Care Reform

The biggest failure of our private-based health insurance system is undoubtedly its failure to provide health coverage for 46 million Americans.[16] The United States can surely afford to insure all its citizens. After all, most European countries, Canada, and Japan, have universal health coverage. One way to increase access to health coverage is to make it illegal for private insurance companies to deny coverage based on pre-existing medical conditions. To prevent insurance companies from charging "undesirable" subscribers high premiums—like the real estate agent who faced a premium of $25,000 *after* being successfully treated for cancer—community rating must be required. With community rating, everybody pays the same premium in a geographic area, thereby spreading the risk of health care costs across a population.

Secondly, the government needs to provide affordable health coverage for people who cannot afford to pay the high premiums. The government could offer a subsidy or tax credit to low-income people buying health insurance in the private market. But with average annual health insurance premiums of $4,824 for individual coverage and $13,375 for family coverage, this is an enormously expensive solution.[17] Alternatively, the government could expand Medicare or offer some other public plan. The costs of covering an individual under a public plan would be substantially lower because the administrative cost of Medicare is less than a third of the administrative cost of private insurance companies.[18]

Although a public health insurance plan like Medicare addresses the issue of high administrative costs, it does not effectively deal with issues of waste and fraud because it keeps the current incentive structures intact. In today's health care system, health care decisions are increasingly influenced by monetary considerations. But monetary considerations are not necessarily in alignment with the interest of the patient, resulting in patients receiving substandard care. The solution is to take the money out of the system.

A first step would be to do away with fee-for-service medicine, where health care providers are paid a fee for each service they provide. The existence of fee-for-service has created a huge bureaucracy paralleling that of the Soviet Union's five-year plans. Furthermore, fee-for-service encourages health care providers to engage in overtreating, overcharging, upcoding, and other fraudulent practices because there is a strong financial incentive to do so. Doctors' practices and hospitals have large billing departments that are responsible for collecting payments from patients and their insurance companies. Disputed claims are shuffled back and forth between billing departments and insurance companies for months. And although it makes economic sense for both health care providers and insurance companies to engage in paper shuffling, it is a waste of economic resources that could be better spent on patient care.

One government program that has taken a very different approach to the remuneration of health care providers is the veteran's health care program.[19] The Veterans Health Administration (VHA) covers 5.6 million veterans and operates 1,400 hospitals, community-based outpatient clinics, and nursing homes.[20] Its 14,800 physicians and 61,000 nurses are paid a salary, and outpatient clinics and hospitals are allocated money at the beginning of each year.

There are no rewards for increasing patient volume by shortening consultation time, performing medically unnecessary surgeries, repeating tests, or prescribing the latest and most expensive drugs instead of the preferable drug. Hospitals that improve safety and quality of care are financially rewarded, as opposed to hospitals in the private sector that are rewarded by treating patients who acquired infections and injuries while under their care.

So, does the different incentive structure of VHA translate into better outcomes? A 2004 study compared the quality of care VA patients received to the care received by patients with similar medical conditions in the private health care sector. The study found that for the 348 measures of quality "the VHA performed consistently better across the entire spectrum of care, including screening, diagnosis, treatment, and follow-up."[21]

Expanding the veteran's health program to nonveterans would mean a *fundamental* reform of the delivery and remuneration of health care services. However, it is not necessary for doctor practices, clinics, and hospitals to be publicly owned as is the case with the VHA; nor need they be owned by a public corporation, as is the case in Great Britain. Doctors' practices, clinics, and hospitals can continue to be privately owned. What must change is the way we reward health care providers. We must shift our focus away from maximizing revenues and toward maximizing quality of care. Only a universal public health care plan can effectively do that.

Private health insurance companies have no financial incentives to invest in prevention and screening because they are unlikely to reap the benefits many years out. Because employers often change the health plan(s) they offer in the quest to lower premiums and because employees change jobs, private health insurance companies have a constant turnover of members. This makes private insurance companies take a short-term view of the benefits that derive from prevention. From a private health insurance company's perspective, the benefits of heart disease prevention are small, for an individual with a high cholesterol level will in all likelihood have left the plan before developing coronary heart disease. As a result, half of adult Americans do not receive the recommended preventive care for their age group.[22]

In a public health care system in which patients have long-standing coverage, prevention of diseases is a good investment. Screening for cancers saves money because treatment of early-stage cancer is cheaper and more successful than late-stage treatment. Management of diabetes is a good investment because eventually complications become expensive. Aggressive treatment of diseases like Lyme disease is a no-brainer because years of therapy for chronic Lyme disease, or post–Lyme disease syndrome, or whatever label the condition is given, is hundreds-fold more expensive.

But what about rationing? A big fuss has been made in the American media about rationing in European public health care systems. Yet rationing is already taking place in the American system to a much greater degree than in Europe; it is just getting little media attention. Rationing essentially means controlling the distribution of scarce goods and services when demand exceeds supply. This means that when your health plan is not covering a medically necessary procedure, it is rationing you. When your health plan has quantity restrictions on prescription drugs, it is rationing you. When you have to wait one month for an appointment with a new in-network physician, it is rationing you. When you don't have health coverage and you cannot afford

care, economists refer to it as "price rationing." Price rationing is
the worst form of rationing, as it is not based on medical needs but
rather on financial means. If you don't have the financial means to
pay for uncovered health care, there is no waiting list you can be
placed on that guarantees you coverage three months out.

Finally, a public health care system should not replace our current system—it should be offered as an alternative. This broadens
Americans' choices in health care. People who want and can afford
to go outside the public program should be able to do so, but their
care should not be subsidized by taxpayers' money because that is a
terrible use of our tax dollars. Arnold Relman, a professor with the
Harvard Medical School, estimates that as much as 40 to 45 percent
of total health care expenditures in the private health sector are
diverted from patient care to unnecessary overhead, marketing, and
advertisement; wasted on unneeded or ineffective medical procedures; paid out as profits; or simply lost to fraud and abuse in billing
practices.[23] That same 40 to 45 percent could be spent on covering
the uninsured and underinsured under a public plan, investing in
prevention, and increasing the quality of care for all Americans.

The United States is the richest country in the world. We have
some of the most highly skilled doctors and have adopted the latest technology; still, a majority of Americans do not receive the
best health care in the world. A lack of money is not the problem.
Americans spend over $2.5 *trillion* on health care a year.[24] The
problem is that our health care system is broken. Specifically, it is
terribly inefficient in allocating economic resources, which results
in waste, high costs, and poor outcomes. The fact that the United
States ranked dead last in preventable deaths among industrialized countries is predictable given our current health care system,
which, by design, does not prioritize quality of care.

By restructuring our health care system, we can change the incentive structures to focus efforts and resources on providing the best care. We know what the underlying problems are. We know how to fix them. Health care reform has the public support, but is there the political will to do it?

Epilogue

In the first year of his presidency, President Obama made health insurance reform one of his top priorities. The main objective of his proposed plan was to provide universal coverage for all Americans. The president's plan would expand private health insurance by prohibiting discrimination based on pre-existing conditions. The president also proposed a public plan as a mechanism to provide competition to private insurers. Described as health *insurance* reform by the president, rather than *health care* reform, the plan did not propose changes to how health care is provided or to the incentive structure of health care providers.

The strength of the plan was that it did not propose major reform. But this was also its weakness. Cost control measures were limited to expanding prevention, reducing waste and fraud, and broadening the use of electronic medical record keeping. Otherwise, the plan did little to contain the rapidly raising costs of health care. In June of 2009, the Congressional Budget Office (CBO) determined the costs of extending coverage to 39 million Americans under the president's plan to be $1 trillion over the next 10 years. To put that number in perspective, consider this: Total annual health care expenditures are projected to be $2.6

trillion in 2010. The total federal government budget in the fiscal year of 2010 is $3.6 trillion. The government has spent more than $900 billion on the wars in Iraq and Afghanistan.

The compromise was to scale back the "universality" of the plan. Another compromise considered relates to how to insure the uninsured. Private health insurance companies lobbied hard against the proposed public plan, fearing that it would provide better health care coverage at a lower cost. Private health insurance companies claimed that they were so uncompetitive, a public plan would force them out of business, as subscribers unhappy with their current private plan would buy into the new public plan. Instead of a public plan, private insurance companies want the government to subsidize private coverage—a very expensive compromise that would increase the costs of health insurance reform considerably, making our unaffordable health care system even more unaffordable.

Despite loud protest from a small minority who tried to drown out the voice of the majority at town hall meetings, public support for health reform is broad—three out of every five Americans support health care reform.[1] Americans generally do not trust health insurance companies, and the majority supports a public option—65 percent according to a CBS News/*New York Times* poll and 55 percent by an ABC News/*Washington Post* poll.[2] Fully 82 percent of Americans support expanding current state programs such as Medicaid and SCHIP to more people.[3] And it is not only patients who want health care reform: 73 percent of physicians favor a public option to be included as a component of expanding health coverage.[4]

The reality is that private health insurance companies have failed to provide insurance, and as a result 46 million Americans are without health insurance coverage. But even people like me, who have health insurance, find that their insurance is pathetically inadequate when they become sick. For years, private insurance companies have claimed that chronic or persistent Lyme disease does not exist and have denied coverage for treatment beyond one month of antibiotics, dooming thousands of Lyme patients to a life of illness.

In July 2009, a hearing was held on the Infectious Diseases Society of America's (IDSA) corrupted guidelines written for health insurance companies.[5] Lorraine Johnson, chief executive officer for the California Lyme Disease Association (CALDA) presented survey data showing that my experience with Lyme disease is far from unique. Fifty-eight percent of respondents said that they remained ill after being treated under the IDSA restrictive guidelines; of these respondents, 60 percent reported improvement with additional courses of antibiotics. Dr. Raphael Stricker, a renowned Lyme disease specialist, gave an overview of the medical literature showing high failure rates of IDSA-recommended treatment. Dr. Kenneth Liegner described the cases of two patients who died from Lyme disease after being denied further treatment. Allison Delong, a biostatistician with Brown University, provided a statistical analysis of the New England Medical Center (NEMC) study on which the IDSA had based its recommendations. Delong found that the NEMC study suffered from "substantial statistical problems that prevent its use in formulating treatment guidelines." The science is clear: two studies found that patients improved with additional therapy, one discredited study found no effect. Presenter after presenter provided scientific validation to what I already knew—that Lyme disease is a serious disease that can destroy your life. The infection can be hard to treat, and in my case required years of therapy.

But with treatment I did get better. It has been a year since

I stopped antibiotic therapy, and this time I have not relapsed. I am driving a car, volunteering at the local Humane Society, and over the summer I worked as an economic consultant. I am not fully recovered. I still have muscle twitching in my face, my brain is working at about half the speed it worked at before my illness, I can't remember from my nose to my mouth as my mother would say, and fatigue continues to slow me down. I don't mind. These are just minor inconveniences. I don't know what my latest test results will show. But I hope that they are negative and that my doctor will tell me, "You are cured!"

Acknowledgments

My deep thanks go to my Lyme friends, Tondia Burrows and Stacey Belyea, who provided great support and encouragement during my illness. Their comments and insights on health insurance coverage issues and Lyme disease were invaluable to the writing of this book. Dr. Sarah Gammage had great confidence from the very beginning in my abilities to write this book, long before anyone else did, including myself. Without her cheerleading, I would never have dared to take on this writing project during the darkest days of my illness.

These people helped me think clearly about the economics of health care and health care reform: Dr. John Schmitt, economist with the Center for Economic and Policy Research; Dr. Lauren Appelbaum, codirector of the Center for Women and Work, Rutgers University; and Dr. Heather Boushey, senior economist with the Joint Economic Committe of the U.S. Congress.

Monte Skall, executive director of the National Capital Lyme and Tick-Borne Disease Association provided insightful comments on the debate over treatment of Lyme disease; Lauren Shababb gave detailed comments on my manuscript; Dr. Virginia Rutter taught me everything I know about book promotion and marketing; and Dr. Daniel Teich, DVM, introduced me to the intriguing world of laboratory and pharmacy pricing. Thank you for your invaluable help.

To my husband, Dean, thank you for your loving support during my illness and your critical review of my writings.

Finally, a special thanks to all the Lyme-literate physicians from whose research and knowledge I have personally benefited tremendously. Without my own physicians' extensive expertise and deep compassion, I would have been doomed to a life of illness without any hope of recovery. Because of their care, I have been able to reclaim my life and write this book.

APPENDIX

Symptoms of Lyme disease

Early stage

Erythema migrans (EM) rash
Fatigue
Chills
Fever
Headache
Muscle ache
Joint aches
Swollen lymph nodes

Intermediate stage

Severe headaches
Neck stiffness
Meningitis
Shooting pains
Heart palpitations
Dizziness
Joint pain and swelling
Bell's palsy (loss of facial
     muscle tone)

Late stage

Arthritis (severe joint pain)
Neurological pain
Numbness
Tingling in hands or feet
Inability to concentrate
Memory loss
Sleep disturbances
Night sweats
Sore throat
Myalgia
Abdominal pain and nausea
Diarrhea
Irritability and mood swings
Depression
Back pain
Blurred vision and eye pain
Testicular/pelvic pain
Tinnitus
Vertigo
Cranial nerve disturbance (facial
     numbness, pain, tingling)
And symptoms from the earlier
     stages of the disease

Sources: Centers for Disease Control and Prevention 2008; Cameron et al. 2006;
Wormser et al. 2006. *Note*: There may be an overlap in the three stages as the
progression of the disease varies across patients.

References

Abelson, Reed. 2006. The spine as profit center. *New York Times,* December 30.

——. 2008. Financial ties are cited as issue in spine study. *New York Times,* January 30.

Adelson, Martin E., Raja-Venkitesh S. Rao, Richard C. Tilton, et al. 2004. Prevalence of *Borrelia burgdorferi, Bartonella* spp., *Babesia microti,* and *Anaplasma phagocytophila* in *Ixodes scapularis* ticks collected in Northern New Jersey. *Journal of Clinical Microbiology* 42(6): 2799–2801.

Alcindor, Yamiche. 2009. A critical situation for area hospitals. *Washington Post,* July 13.

American College of Physicians. 1997. Guidelines for laboratory evaluation in the diagnosis of Lyme disease. *Annals of Internal Medicine* 127(12): 1106–8.

American Hospital Association. 2001. Patients or paperwork: The regulatory burden facing America's hospitals. Report, May.

Anderson, Jenny. 2005. Today's insider trading suspect may wear a lab coat. *New York Times,* August 9.

Anderson, Liz. 2006. Dozens from Dutchess join Lyme treatment rally. *The Journal News,* December 1.

Appleby, June. 2008. As drug ads surge, more get Rx's filled. *USA Today,* March 4.

Arrow, Kenneth J. 1963. Uncertainty and the welfare economics of medical care. *American Economic Review* 53(5): 941–73.

Asch, Steven M., Elizabeth A. McGlynn, Mary M. Hogan, et al. 2004. Comparison of quality for patients in the Veteran's Health Administration and patients in a national sample. *Annals of Internal Medicine* 141(12): 938–45.

Association of American Medical Colleges. 2009. Financial planning: How much does medical school cost and can I afford it? www.aamc .org/students/financing/start.htm.

Bakken, Lori L, Kay L. Case, Steven M. Callister, et al. 1992. Performance of 45 laboratories participating in a proficiency testing problem for Lyme disease serology. *JAMA* 268(7): 891–5.

Berenson, Alex, and Reed Abelson. 2008. Weighing the costs of a CT scan's look inside the heart. *New York Times*, June 29.

Blake, Robert L., and E. K. Early. 1995. Patients' attitudes about gifts to physicians from pharmaceutical companies. *Journal of American Board of Family Practice* 8(6): 457–64.

Bogdanich, Walt. 2008a. The drug scare that exposed a world of hurt. *New York Times*, March 30.

———. 2008b. Heparin discovery may point to Chinese counterfeiting. *New York Times*, March 20.

Bond, C. A., Cynthia L. Raehl, Michael E. Pitterle, and Todd Franke. 1999. Health care professional staffing, hospital characteristics, and hospital mortality rates. *Pharmacotherapy* 19(2): 130–8.

Brennan, Troyen A., David J. Rothman, Linda Blank, et al. 2006. Health industry practices that create conflicts of interest. *JAMA* 295(4): 429–30.

Brody, Howard. 2005. The company we keep: Why physicians should refuse to see pharmaceutical representatives. *Annals of Family Medicine* 3(1): 82–5.

Brorson, Oystein, and Sverre-Henning Brorson. 1997. Transformation of cystic forms of *Borrelia burgdorferi* to normal, mobile spirochetes. *Infection* 25(4): 240–6.

Bureau of Labor Statistics (BLS). 2009. Employee benefits in the United States, March 2009. News release, July 28.

Burgdorfer, Willy, Alan G. Barbour, Stanley F. Hayes, Jorge L. Benach, Edgar Grunwaldt, and Jeffrey P. Davis. 1982. Lyme disease—a tick-borne spirochetosis? *Science* 216: 1317–9.

Cameron, Daniel, Andrea Gaito, Nick Harris, et al. 2004. Evidence-based guidelines for the management of Lyme disease. *Expert Review of Anti-Infective Therapy* 2(1): S1–S13.

Casalino, Lawrence P., Daniel Dunham, Marshall H. Chin, et al. 2009. Frequency of failure to inform patients of clinically significant outpatient test results. *Archives of Internal Medicine* 169(12): 1123–9.

Casjens, Sherwood, N. Palmer, Richard van Vugt, et al. 2000. A bacterial genome in flux: The twelve linear and nice circular extrachromosomal

DNAs in an infectious isolate of the Lyme disease spirochete *Borrelia burgdorferi*. *Molecular Microbiology* 35(3): 490–516.

Centers for Disease Control and Prevention (CDC). 2004. Lyme disease—United States, 2001–2002. *Morbidity and Mortality Weekly Report* 53(17): 365–9.

———. 2008. Lyme disease: Lyme disease treatment and prognosis. Division of Vector-Borne Infectious Diseases. www.cdc.gov/ncidod/dvbid/lyme/ld_humandisease_treatment.htm.

———. 2009a. Babesiosis. Division of Parasitic Diseases. www.dpd.cdc.gov/dpdx/HTML/Babesiosis.htm.

———. 2009b. Reported Lyme disease cases by state, 1999–2008. www.cdc.gov/ncidod/dvbid/lyme/resources/ReportedCasesLymeDisease99-2008.pdf.

Centers for Medicare and Medicaid Services (CMS). 2007. Medicare program; changes to the hospital inpatient prospective payment. Final Rule. 42CFR parts 411, 412, 413 and 489. *Federal Register*, August 1.

———. 2009. *National Health Expenditures (NHE) Projections 2008-2018; Forecast Summary and Selected Tables*. Washington DC: U.S. Department of Health and Human Services, February.

Cleveland Clinic. 2008. Cleveland Clinic makes physician disclosures available online. News release, December 3, 2008.

Commonwealth Fund. 2008. Why not the best: Results from the national scorecard on U.S. health system performance, 2008. Report by the Commonwealth Fund Commission on a High Performance Health System, July.

Congressional Budget Office (CBO). 2006. Research and development in the pharmaceutical industry. Report, October.

Connecticut Attorney General's Office, State of Connecticut. 2008. Attorney general's investigation reveals flawed Lyme disease process, IDSA agrees to reassess guidelines, instate independent arbiter. Press release, May 1. www.ct.gov/ag/cwp/view.asp?a=2795&q=414284.

Consumer Reports. 2007. Free drug samples have hidden drawbacks. *ConsumerReports.org*, August.

Cunningham, Peter J. 2008. Trade-offs getting tougher: Problems paying medical bills increase for U.S. families, 2003–2007. Tracking report no. 21, September.

Das, Subrata, Gautam Banerjee, Kathleen DePonte, Nancy Marcantonio, Fred S. Kantor, and Erol Fikrig. 2001. Salp25D, an *Ixodes scapularis* antioxidant, is 1 of 14 immunodominant antigens in engorged tick salivary glands. *Journal of Infectious Diseases* 184: 1056–64.

Dattwyler, Raymond J., John J. Halperin, David J. Volkman, and Benjamin J. Luft. 1988. Treatment of late Lyme borreliosis—randomized comparison of ceftriaxone and penicillin. *Lancet* 1(8596): 1191–4.

DeCarlo, Scott. 2005. CEO Compensation. *Forbes Magazine*, special report, April 21.

Depietropaolo, Daniel L., John H. Powers, James M. Gill, and Andrew J. Foy. 2005. Diagnosis of Lyme disease. *American Family Physician* 72(2): 297–304.

Devereaux, P.J., Peter T. Choi, Christina Lacchetti, et al. 2002. A systematic review and meta-analysis of studies comparing mortality rates of private for-profit and private not-for-profit hospitals. *Canadian Medical Association Journal* 166(11): 1399–1405.

Donohue, Julie M., Marisa Cevasco, and Meredith B. Rosenthal. 2007. A decade of direct-to-consumer advertising of prescription drugs. *New England Journal of Medicine* 357(7): 673–81.

Drummond, Roger. 2000. *Ticks and What You Can Do about Them.* Berkeley: Wilderness Press.

Embers, Monica E., Ramesh Ramamoorthy, and Mario T. Philipp. 2004. Survival strategies of *Borrelia burgdorferi*, the etiologic agent of Lyme disease. *Microbes and Infection* 6(3): 312–8.

EUCALB. 2007. Biology: The Tick: Introduction. European Union Concerted Action on Lyme Borreliosis. http://meduni09.edis.at/eucalb/cms/index.php.

Executive Office of the President and the Council of Economic Advisers. 2009. *The Economic Report of the President.* Washington DC: U.S. Government Printing Office.

Fallon, Brian A., John Keilp, Kathy M. Corbera, et al. 2008. A randomized, placebo-controlled trial of repeated IV antibiotic therapy for Lyme encephalopathy. *Neurology* 70(13): 992–1003.

Federal Bureau of Investigation (FBI). 2008. Financial crimes report to the public, fiscal year 2007. www.fbi.gov/publications/financial/fcs_report2007/financial_crime_2007.htm#health.

Federal Trade Commission (FTC). 2002. Generic drug entry prior to patent expiration: A FTC study. Report, July. www.ftc.gov/os/2002/07/genericdrugstudy.pdf.

———. 2006. FTC testifies on barriers to the entry of generic drugs. News release, July 20. www.ftc.gov/opa/2006/07/genericdrug.shtm.

Forelle, Charles, and James Bandler. 2006. The perfect payday. *Wall Street Journal*, March 19.

Forelle, Charles, and Mark Maramont. 2006. UnitedHealth's McGuire could leave with $1.1 billion. *Wall Street Journal*, October 17.

Frank, Richard G. 2007. The ongoing regulation of generic drugs. *New England Journal of Medicine* 357(20): 1993–6.

Freed, Joshua. 2006. UnitedHealthcare's stock options problems. *Associated Press*, October 16.

Freudenheim, Milt. 2004. Merck and Vioxx: The company; a blow to efforts to close in on rivals. *New York Times*, October 1.

———. 2007. A small business, one illness can send insurance costs soaring. *New York Times*, May 5.

———. 2008. Trying to save by increasing doctors' fees. *New York Times*, July 21.

Gardner, Amanda. 2008. FDA: Contaminated heparin found in 11 countries. *Washington Post*, April 22.

Girion, Lisa. 2007. Blue Shield sued over revoked insurance. *Los Angeles Times*, February 16.

———. 2008a. State steps up scrutiny of insurers. *Los Angeles Times*, January 30.

———. 2008b. Major health insurers accused of rigging rates. *Los Angeles Times*, February 13.

Golden, Lonnie, and Helene Jorgensen. 2002. Time after time: Mandatory overtime in the U.S. economy. Economic Policy Institute, Briefing paper, January.

Goodman, David C., and Elliott S. Fisher. 2008. Physician workforce crisis? Wrong diagnosis, wrong prescription. *New England Journal of Medicine* 358(16): 1658–61.

Government Accountability Office (GAO). 2007. Drug safety: Preliminary findings suggest weakness in FDA's program for inspecting foreign drug manufacturers. Testimony before the Subcommittee on Oversight and Investigations, Committee on Energy and Commerce, House of Representatives, November 1.

Greider, Katharine. 2003. *The Big Fix: How the Pharmaceutical Industry Rips Off American Consumers*. New York: Public Affairs.

Hakim, Danny, and Reed Abelson. 2009. Big health insurer agrees to update its fee data. *New York Times*, January 13.

Harris, Gardiner. 2008a. Top psychiatrist failed to report drug income. *New York Times*, October 4.

———. 2008b. U.S. identifies tainted heparin in 11 countries. *New York Times*, April 22.

Harris, Gardiner, and Walt Bogdanich. 2008. Blood thinner linked to China had contaminant, F.D.A. says. *New York Times*, March 6.

Hartz, A. J., H. Krakauer, E. M. Kuhn, et al. 1989. Hospital characteristics and mortality rates. *New England Journal of Medicine* 321(25): 1720–5.

HealthGrades. 2008. Medical error cost U.S. $8.8 billion, result in 238,337 potentially preventable deaths, according the HealthGrades study. News release, April 8.

Hedayati, Tarlan, and Joseph Choi. 2009. Babesiosis. *Emedicine from WebMD*, April 28. www.emedicine.com/emerg/topic49.htm.

———. 2009a. More than half of Americans say family skimped on medical care because of cost in the past year; worries about affordability and availability of care rise. News release, February 25.

Henry J. Kaiser Family Foundation. 2009b. *Employer Health Benefits: 2009 Annual Survey.* Menlo Park: Kaiser Family Foundation, September.

———. 2009c. Public support for health reform increases in September, reversing summer declines as Congress takes up legislation. News Release, September 29.

Hodzic, Emir, Sunlian Feng, Kevin Holden, Kimberly J. Freet, and Stephen W. Barthold. 2008. Persistence of *Borrelia burgdorferi* following antibiotic treatment in mice. *Antimicrobial Agents and Chemotherapy* 52(5): 1728–36.

Kaufman, Marc. 2008a. Contaminant in heparin is identified. *Washington Post*, March 20.

———. 2008b. FDA says it approved the wrong drug plant. *Washington Post*, February 19.

Keirans, Jim E., H. J. Hutcheson, Lance A. Durden, and Johan S. Klompen. 1996. *Ixodes* (*Ixodes*) *scapularis* (*Acari*: *Ixodidae*): Redescription of all active stages, distribution, hosts, geographical variation, and medical and veterinary importance. *Journal of Medical Entomology* 33(3): 297–318.

Keyhani, Salomeh, and Alex Federman. 2009. Doctors on coverage— physicians' views on a new public insurance option and Medicare expansion. *New England Journal of Medicine*, September 14. http://healthcarereform.nejm.org/?p=1790#printpreview.

Kirkpatrick, David D. 2005a. Senate leader explains his sale of a stock that then plummeted. *New York Times*, September 22.

———. 2005b. Agency calls on Frist about timing of stock sale. *New York Times*, September 23.

Klempner, Mark S., Linden T. Hu, Janine Evans, et al. 2001. Two controlled trials of antibiotic treatment in patients with persistent symptoms and a history of Lyme disease. *New England Journal of Medicine* 345: 85–92.

Klevens, R. Monina, Jonathan R. Edwards, Chesley L. Richards, et al. 2007. Estimating health care–associated infection and deaths in U.S. hospitals, 2002. *Public Health Reports* 122: 160–6.

Kolata, Gina. 2008. Citing ethics, some doctors are rejecting industry pay. *New York Times*, April 15, Science section.

Krause, Peter J., Sam R. Telford, Andrew Spielman, et al. 1996. Concurrent Lyme disease and babesiosis. Evidence for increased severity and duration of illness. *JAMA* 275(21): 1657–60.

Krupp, Lauren B., Leslie G. Hyman, Roger Grimson, et al. 2003. Study and treatment of post–Lyme disease (STOP-LD): A randomized double masked clinical trial. *Neurology* 60: 1923–30.

Kuthejlova, Marie, Jan Kopecky, Gabriela Stepanova, and Ales Macela. 2001. Tick salivary gland extract inhibits killing of *Borrelia afzelii* spirochetes by mouse macrophages. *Infection and Immunity* 69(1): 575–8.

Kuttner, Robert. 2008. Market-based failure—A second opinion on U.S. health care costs. *New England Journal of Medicine* 358(6): 549–51.

Levine, Susan. 2007a. Bug puts hospitals on edge, on guard. *Washington Post*, May 14.

———. 2007b. D.C. hospital in critical condition, City officials told. *Washington Post*, May 24.

Logigian, Eric L., Richard F. Kaplan, and Allen C. Steere. 1990. Chronic neurologic manifestations of Lyme disease. *New England Journal of Medicine* 323(21): 1438–44

———. 1999. Successful treatment of Lyme encephalopathy with intravenous ceftriaxone. *Journal of Infectious Diseases* 180: 377–83.

Longman, Phillip. 2007. *Best Care Anywhere: Why VA Health Care Is Better Than Yours*. Sausalito, CA: PoliPointPress.

Luger, Steven W., and Elliot Krauss. 1990. Serologic tests for Lyme disease. Interlaboratory variability. *Archives of Internal Medicine* 150(4): 761–3.

Lyme Disease Association. 2008. LymeRPrimer. www.lymedisease association.org/LymeRPrimer.pdf.

Marshall, W. F., Sam R. Telford, Paul N. Rys, et al. 1994. Detection of *Borrelia burgdorferi* DNA in museum specimens of *Peromyscus leucopus*. *Journal of Infectious Diseases* 170(4): 1027–32.

Mayo, Rachel. 2006. Veteran's Health Administration: The best value in healthcare. Report HS 6000, December 15.

McCoy, J. J. 2003. Amy Tan, ticked off about Lyme. *Washington Post*, August 5, Health Section.

McGuire, Steven. 2007. Pfizer settles with Novatis in Zithromax lawsuit. *Medical Marketing and Media News Online*, July 6.

McKay, Niccie L., Christy H. Lemak, Annesha Lovett, and R. Roy Wright. 2008. Variation in hospital administrative costs. *Journal of Healthcare Management*, May 1.

Medical Group Management Association (MGMA). 2009. Physician compensation and production survey: 2009 report based on 2008 data. www.mgma.com/WorkArea/mgma_downloadasset .aspx?id=29312

Melia, Michael. 2007. Pharmaceutical plants retreat from PR. *Associated Press*, November 18.

Merriam, Ginny. 2004. Health officials search for illness as warm weather brings out ticks. *Missoulian.com—Western Montana's News Online*, March 30.

Mishori, Ranit. 2009. Don't let a hospital make you sick. *Parade Magazine*, February 8.

Montgomery, Ruth R., Denise Lusitani, Anne B. Chevance, and Stephen E. Malawista. 2004. Tick saliva reduces adherence and area of human neutrophils. *Infection and Immunity* 72(5): 2989–94.

Montgomery, Ruth R., Kimberly Schreck, Xiaomei Wang, and Stephen E. Malawista. 2006. Human neutrophil calprotectin reduces the susceptibility of *Borrelia burgdorferi* to penicillin. *Infection and Immunity* 74(4): 2468–72.

Mukherjee, Debabrata, Steven E. Nissen, and Eric J. Topol. 2001. Risk of cardiovascular events associated with selective COX-2 inhibitors. *JAMA* 286(8): 954–9.

Nakamura, David. 2007. City, buyers reach deal on Southeast hospital. *Washington Post*, September 17.

Nakamura, David, and Susan Levine. 2007. D.C. mayor warms to offer to sell hospital. *Washington Post*, August 24.

Nagourney, Adam, and Dalia Sussman. 2009. In poll, public wary of Obama on war and health. *New York Times*, September 25.

National Health Care Anti-Fraud Association. 2008. The problem of health care fraud. Consumer alert. www.nhcaa.org/eweb/Dynamic Page.aspx?webcode=anti_fraud_resource_centr&wpscode=The ProblemOfHCFraud.

National Institute for Health Care Management. 2002. Changing patterns of pharmaceutical innovation. Report.

National Library of Medicine. 2006. Historic medical sites in the Washington DC area: 3. District of Columbia General Hospital.

Bethesda, MD: National Institutes of Health. www.nlm.nih.gov/
hmd/medtour/dcgeneral.html.

National Women's Health Network and Pharmedout.org. 2007. Fast
facts on generic drugs. Fact sheet, December. www.pharmedout.org/
FastFactsGenerics.pdf.

Nery, Steve. 2006. Lyme disease patients to protest new guidelines. *Star
Democratic*, November 26.

New York Times. (Letter to the editor) 1919. Failing medical schools:
Shortage of physicians will make itself felt a few years hence. July 20.

New York Times. Editorial. 2009. Not so reasonable and customary.
January 17.

Nguyen, Quoc V. 2009. Hospital-acquired infections. Emedicine,
WebMD, January 14.

Nolte, Ellen, and C. Martin McKee. 2008. Measuring the health of
nations: Updating an earlier analysis. *Health Affairs* 27(1): 58–71.

Oksi, Jarmo, Jukka Nikoskelainen, and Matti K. Viljanen. 1998. Comparison of oral cefixime and intravenous ceftriaxone followed by oral
amoxicillin in disseminated Lyme borreliosis. *European Journal of
Clinical Microbiology and Infectious Diseases* 17(10): 715–9.

Organisation for Economic Co-Operation and Development (OECD).
2009. OECD health data 2009—Frequently requested data, June.
www.oecd.org/document/16/0,3343,en_2649_34631_2085200_1
_1_1_1,00.html.

Ornstein, Charles. 2002. Kaiser clerks paid more for helping less. *Los
Angeles Times*, May 17.

Pear, Robert. 2007. Without health benefits, a good life turns fragile.
New York Times, March 5.

Pearlstein, Steven. 2007. Hospitals check their charts. *Washington Post*,
April 20.

Pharmaceutical Research and Manufacturers of America (PhRMA).
2007. R&D spending by U.S. biopharmaceutical companies reaches a
record $55.2 billion in 2006. News release, February 12.

Poon, Eric G., Tejal K. Gandhi, Thomas D. Sequist, Harvey J. Murff,
Andrew S. Karson, and David W. Bates. 2004. "I wish I had seen this
test result earlier!" Dissatisfaction with test result management systems in primary care. *Archives of Internal Medicine*, 164(20): 2223–8.

Porcella, Stephen F., and Tom G. Schwan. 2001. *Borrelia burgdorferi* and
Treponema pallidum: A comparison of functional genomics, environ-
mental adaptations, and pathogenic mechanisms. *Journal of Clinical
Investigation* 107(6): 651–6.

Quick, Robert E., Barbara L. Herwaldt, John W. Thomford, et al. 1993.

Babesiosis in Washington State: A new species of *Babesia*? *Annals of Internal Medicine* 119(4): 284–90.

Rabin, Roni C. 2007. Free drug samples? Bad idea, some say. *New York Times,* May 1. Science section.

Rein, Lisa. 2009. Hospitals tally their avoidable mistakes. *Washington Post,* July 21.

Reinberg, Steven. 2008. Mix-up behind FDA's failure to inspect China blood-thinner plant. *Washington Post,* February 18.

Relman, Arnold S. 2007. *A Second Opinion: Rescuing America's Health Care.* New York: PublicAffairs, A Century Foundation Book.

Ribeiro, Jose M., and Ivo M. Francischetti. 2003. Role of arthropod saliva in blood feeding. *Annual Review of Entomology* 48(1): 73–88.

Robbins, Jim. 2003. Montana lab tries to identify tick-borne disease. *New York Times,* May 20.

Ruzic-Sabljic, Eva, Tjasa Podreka, Vera Maraspin, and Franc Strle. 2005. Susceptibility of *Borrelia afzelii* strains to antimicrobial agents. *International Journal of Antimicrobial Agents* 25(6): 474–8.

Sack, Kevin. 2007. Swabs in hand, hospital cuts deadly infections. *New York Times,* July 27.

———. 2008. In Massachusetts, universal coverage strains care. *New York Times,* April 5.

Saul, Stephanie. 2005. Gimme an Rx! Cheerleaders pep up drug sales. *New York Times,* November 28.

Schoen, Cathy, Sara R. Collins, Jennifer L. Kriss, and Michelle M. Doty. 2008. How many are underinsured? Trends among U.S. adults, 2003 and 2007. *Health Affairs* 27(4): w298–w309.

Schumann, Richard E. 2001. Compensation from World War II through the Great Society. *Compensation and Working Conditions,* fall issue.

Shahpoori, Karen P., and James Smith. 2005. Wages in profit and nonprofit hospitals and universities. Bureau of Labor Statistics, June. www.bls.gov/opub/cwc/print/cm20050624ar01p1.htm.

Siegel, Jane D., Emily Rhinehart, Marguerite Jackson, Linda Chiarello. 2006. Management of multidrug-resistant organisms in health care settings, 2006. Guidelines published by the Centers for Disease Control and Prevention, October 19.

Silverman, Elaine M., Jonathan S. Skinner, and Elliott S. Fisher. 1999. The association between for-profit hospital ownership and increased Medicare spending. *New England Journal of Medicine* 341(6): 420–6.

Stanglin, Douglas. 2007. Audit: FDA hampered in review of imported drugs. *USA Today,* November 1.

Steinbrook, Robert. 2008. Health care reform in Massachusetts— Expanding coverage, escalating costs. *New England Journal of Medicine* 358(26): 2757–60.

Stolberg, Sheryl G. 2005. For Frist, a political fortune may be inextricably linked to a financial one. *New York Times*, October 25.

Straubinger, Reinhard K., Alix F. Straubinger, Brian A. Summers, Richard H. Jacobson, and Hollis N. Erb. 1998. Clinical manifestation, pathogenesis, and effect of antibiotic treatment on Lyme borreliosis in dogs. *Wiener Klinische Wochenschrift* 110: 874–81.

Stricker, Raphael B. 2006. Controversies in Lyme disease: Diagnosis and treatment. Presentation at the Infectious Diseases Society of American Annual Meetings, Toronto, Ontario, Canada, October 12.

Symm, Barbalee, Michael Averitt, Samuel N. Forjuoh, and Cheryl Preece. 2006. Effects of using free sample medications on the prescribing practices of family physicians. *Journal of American Board of Family Medicine* 19(5): 443–9.

Tanne, Janice H. 2002. Mortality higher at for-profit hospitals. *British Medical Journal* 324: 1351.

Tarkan, Laurie. 2002. Blood-test labs bypass doctors, spurring debate. *New York Times*, March 12.

Theodosakis, Jason, and David T. Feinberg. 2000. *Don't Let Your HMO Kill You: How to Wake Up Your Doctor, Take Control of Your Health, and Make Managed Care Work for You*. New York: Routledge.

Thomas, Venetta, Juan Anguita, Stephen W. Barthold, and Erol Fikrig. 2001. Coinfection with *Borrelia burgdorferi* and the agent of human granulocytic ehrlichiosis alters murine immune responses, pathogen burden, and severity of Lyme arthritis. *Infection and Immunity* 69(5): 3359–71.

Timmerman, Luke, and David Heath. 2005. Drug researchers leak secrets to Wall St. *Seattle Times*, August 7.

Topol, Eric J. 2004. Good riddance to a bad drug. *New York Times*, October 2. Op-ed.

Topol, Eric J., and David Blumenthal. 2005. Physicians and the investment industry. *JAMA* 293(21): 2654–7.

Treib, Johannes, A. Fernandez, Anton Haass, Markus T. Grauer, Georg Holzer, and Ralph Woessner. 1998. Clinical and serologic follow-up in patients with neuroborreliosis. *Neurology* 51(5): 1489–91.

Tufts Managed Care Institute. 1998. A brief history of managed care. www.thci.org/downloads/briefhist.pdf.

Tugwell, Peter, David T. Dennis, Arthur Weinstein, et al. 1997. Laboratory evaluation in the diagnosis of Lyme disease. *Annals of Internal Medicine* 127(12): 1109–23.

U.S. Census Bureau. 2009a. *Income, Poverty, and Health Insurance Coverage in the United States: 2008.* Current Population Reports, P60–236. Washington DC: U.S. Government Printing Office, September.

———. 2009b. *Statistical Abstract of the United States 2009.* Washington DC: U.S. Government Printing Office.

U.S. Department of Health and Human Services. 2009. New data say uninsured account for nearly one-fifth of emergency room visits. News release, July 15.

U.S. Department of Justice. 2000. HCA—the health care company and subsidiaries to pay $840 million in criminal fines and civil damages and penalties. Largest government fraud settlement in U.S. history. Press release, December 14. www.usdoj.gov/opa/pr/2000/december/696civcrm.

U.S. Department of the Treasurer. 2008. Treasury, IRS issue 2009 indexed amounts for health savings accounts. Press release, May 13.

U.S. Fish and Wildlife Service (FWS). 2001. Carnivore biology/safety. Living with Carnivores Workshop in Idaho, July.

U.S. Food and Drug Administration (FDA). 2004. Risk of acute myocardial infraction and sudden cardiac death in patients treated with COX-2 selective and non-selective NSAIDs. Memorandum from David J. Graham, MD, MPH, associate director of science, Office of Drug Safety to Paul Seligman, MD, MPH, acting director, Office of Drug Safety, September 30. www.fda.gov/CDER/DRUG/infopage/vioxx/vioxxgraham.phf.

U.S. Security and Exchange Commission (SEC). 2007. Former United-Health Group CEO/chairman settles stock options backdating case for $468 million. News release, December 6.

Vredevoe, Larisa. (Year unknown.) Background information on the biology of ticks. Department of Entomology, University of California, Davis, California. http://entomology.ucdavis.edu/faculty/rbkimsey/bickbio.html.

Wahlberg, Peter, Hans Granlund, Dag Nyman, Jaana Panelius, and Iikka Seppala. 1994. Treatment of late Lyme borreliosis. *Journal of Infection* 29(3): 255–61.

Washington Post. 2009. Washington Post—ABC News poll, September 13. www.washingtonpost.com/wp-srv/politics/polls/postpoll_091309.html?sid=ST2009091400007.

Weintraub, Pamela. 2008. *Cure Unknown. Inside the Lyme Epidemic.* New York: St. Martin's Press.

Wormser, Gary P., Raymond J. Dattwyler, Eugene D. Shapiro, et al. 2006. The clinical assessment, treatment, and prevention of Lyme disease, human granulocytic anaplasmosis, and babesiosis: Clinical practice guidelines by the Infectious Diseases Society of America. *Clinical Infectious Diseases* 43: 1089–1134.

Ziegler, Michael G., Pauline Lew, and Brian C. Singer. 1995. The accuracy of drug information from pharmaceutical sales representatives. *JAMA* 273(16): 1296–8.

Zwillich, Todd. 2006. New guidelines on hospital infections: CDC calls on hospitals, others to work harder to stop drug-resistant infections. *WebMD Health News*, October 19. www.webmd.com/news/20061019/new-guidelines-on-hospital-infections.

Notes

Chapter 1: Paradise Valley

1. Cunningham 2008: Tables 1, 2.
2. The median medical debt was $1,930 for medical expenses. Twenty-five percent of families owed $4,920 or more in medical debt.
3. Henry J. Kaiser Family Foundation 2009a: Table 1.
4. Centers for Medicare and Medicaid Services 2009: Table 1.
5. Ibid.
6. Executive Office of the President and the Council of Economic Advisers 2009: Tables B-1, B-16.
7. In February 2003, I had an X-ray and an MRI of my knee that had become swollen and inflamed. From the explanation of benefits from my health plan, the list price of the X-ray was $70 and $1,095 for the MRI.
8. Organisation for Economic Co-Operation and Development 2009: Table on total expenditures on health/capita, US$ PPP (purchasing power parity). The OECD uses a slightly different definition of national health care expenditures than the CMS. The OECD's estimate of U.S. health care costs is $7,290 in 2007, which is lower than the estimate by the CMS of $7,420, also in 2007.
9. U.S. Census Bureau 2009a: Table 7. The data on uninsured are for the year 2008. Forty-six million people were without health insurance coverage at one point in time. Many more people went without health insurance at some point during 2008.
10. Schoen et al. 2008. Being underinsured is defined as having out-of-pocket medical expenses of more than 10% of annual family income, or medical expenses equal to 5% or more for low-income families.

Chapter 2: The Insurance Industry

1. The CDC reported the first two cases of Lyme disease in the state of Montana in 2006.

Even though my infection with Lyme disease met the reporting requirements of the CDC, my case was never recorded in the state of Montana or the District of Columbia in April 2003.

2. During the spring of 1990, I had several bouts of high fever, a stiff and painful neck, knee pain, painful throat, and tonsillitis while living in central Massachusetts. The doctors I consulted could not find any cause for my illness, despite extensive testing, but treated it with antibiotics. At no point was Lyme disease mentioned, and my medical reports showed that they never tested for Lyme disease.

3. Girion 2008a.

4. Pear 2007. According to the National Association of Realtors, 28% of its 1.3 million members do not have health insurance coverage.

5. U.S. Census Bureau 2009a: Table 7.

6. U.S. Census Bureau 2009a: Tables 7, C-1.

7. Kuttner 2008.

8. U.S. Census Bureau 2009a: Table C-1.

9. Bureau of Labor Statistics 2009: Table 2.

10. Henry J. Kaiser Family Foundation 2009b: Exhibits 2.1, 2.2. Almost all companies with 200 or more employees offered health insurance, whereas smaller companies were less likely to offer insurance. About 90 percent of companies with 25 to 49 employees offered health coverage, but only half of companies with fewer than 10 employees did.

11. Henry J. Kaiser Family Foundation 2009b: Exhibits 6.3, 6.4.

12. Bureau of Labor Statistics 2009: Table 2.

13. Freudenheim 2007.

14. Henry J. Kaiser Family Foundation 2009b. Exhibits 6.2, 6.3. Average annual premium for family coverage increased from $5,791 in 1999 to $12,680 in 2008.

15. Bureau of Labor Statistics, 2009: Consumer price index for urban consumers (CPI-U); and median weekly earnings for full-time workers 16 years and older.

16. Organisation for Economic Co-Operation and Development (OECD) 2009; Centers for Medicare and Medicaid Services 2009: Table 1.

17. Theodosakis and Feinberg 2000: 182.

18. Relman 2007: 64.

19. DeCarlo 2005.

20. Henry J. Kaiser Family Foundation 2009b: Exhibits 1.1, 5.1.

21. Hakim and Abelson 2009; Girion 2008b.

22. *New York Times* editorial 2009.

23. Because my health plan negotiated lower charges with providers, the total expenses without insurance is higher than the total medical expenses paid by my plan plus myself.

24. Tufts Managed Care Institute 1998.

25. Kaiser Permanente, About Us. Web site: www.kaiserpermanente .com.

26. Schumann 2001.

27. The Consolidated Omnibus Budget Reconciliation Act of 1986, called COBRA for short, provides the option to continue health care coverage after the termination of employment. Under COBRA, individuals can purchase health insurance from the former employer for up to 18 months, but they have to pay the whole premiums. Most unemployed cannot afford the high insurance premiums. Because people who involuntarily lost their jobs during the economic recession needed help to pay for continued insurance under COBRA, the American Recovery and Reinvestment Act of 2009, also known as the stimulus package, provided a government subsidy of 65 percent of total premiums for nine months.

28. Bureau of Labor Statistics 2009: Table 2. Workers in private industries.

29. Henry J. Kaiser Family Foundation 2009a.

30. U.S. Department of Health and Human Services 2009.

31. Alcindor 2009.

32. Centers for Medicare and Medicaid Services 2009: Table 1.

33. Nolte and Mckee 2008.

Chapter 3: Doctors

1. McCoy 2003.

2. According to the CDC's surveillance guidelines (2008), a bull's-eye rash does not occur in 20 to 30 percent of all patients with Lyme disease. The Lyme Disease Association estimates that less than half of those with Lyme disease have a rash at the bite site (2008).

3. Kuttner 2008.

4. Embers et al. 2004; Montgomery et al. 2006.

5. Thomas et al. 2001.

6. Drummond 2000; Adelson et al. 2004.

7. Krause et al. 1996. Studies on coinfections have found that about

one-third of patients with Lyme disease were coinfected with babesiosis in New England, whereas about a quarter of patients in California were coinfected. About two percent of patients were coinfected with three different tick-borne diseases at the same time. Studies also showed that people coinfected with two or more tick-borne infections were more severely sick, and their illness lasted longer.

8. Robbins 2003; Merriam 2004.

9. Quick et al. 1993. The West Coast strain, WA-1, was officially named *Babesia duncani* in 2006 after the microbiologist J. F. Duncan with the U.S. Naval Medical Research Institute for his research on piroplasms in wild mammals in California in the 1960s.

10. Hedayati and Choi 2009.

11. Centers for Disease Control and Prevention 2009a.

12. Quick et al. 1993.

13. Some antibiotics, such as doxycyline and Flagyl have antiparasitic properties and are used in prevention and treatment of malaria, as well as the treatment of babesiosis.

14. Appleby 2008.

15. Deductible maximum for year 2009.

16. HSA was enacted as part of the Medicare Prescription Drug, Improvement and Modernization Act of 2003.

17. U.S. Department of the Treasurer 2008. Numbers are for 2009. The upper limits increase each year.

18. Henry J. Kaiser Family Foundation 2009b: Exhibit 8.1.

19. Relman 2007.

20. Abelson 2006.

21. Abelson 2008.

22. Abelson 2006; 2008.

23. Timmerman and Heath 2005.

24. Topol and Blumenthal 2005.

25. Timmerman and Heath 2005.

26. Anderson 2005. The Security and Exchange Commission (SEC) subsequently opened investigations into the 26 cases in which physicians sold confidential information from drug trials to insider traders.

27. Kolata 2008.

28. Cleveland Clinic 2008.

29. Harris 2008a.

30. Payments less than $500 would be exempt.

31. Although the 2007 version of the bill died in committee, similar bills have been introduced in both the House and the Senate.

32. Goodman and Fisher 2008: 1660.

33. Relman 2007: 16.

34. Freudenheim 2008.

35. Goodman and Fisher 2008: Table 1.

36. The Massachusetts law exempts employers with 10 or fewer employees.

37. Steinbrook 2008: 2757.

38. Sack 2008.

39. *New York Times* 1919.

40. Association of American Medical Colleges 2009.

41. Medical Group Management Association 2009.

42. Centers for Medicare and Medicaid Services 2009: Table 7.

43. Organisation for Economic Co-Operation and Development 2009.

44. Berenson and Abelson 2008.

45. Commonwealth Fund 2008: 12.

Chapter 4: Drugs

1. Greider 2003: 66.

2. Brody 2005.

3. Saul 2005.

4. Ziegler et al. 1995.

5. *Consumer Reports* 2007. *Consumer Reports* further warns that free drug samples often don't come with printed instructions and warnings about side effects and harmful interactions with other drugs.

6. Symm et al. 2006.

7. Rabin 2007.

8. Greider 2003: 77.

9. Blake and Early 1995.

10. Greider 2003: 82.

11. Brennan et al. 2006.

12. Donohue et al. 2007.

13. Congressional Budget Office 2006: 7. The estimates are based on an analysis by the National Science Foundation. The industry's trade organization, Pharmaceutical Research and Manufacturers of America (PhRMA), estimates that U.S. pharmaceutical and biotechnology companies spent $55.2 billion on research and development worldwide in 2006, but that figure includes research on biotechnology as well as research done in other parts of the world.

14. Frank 2007: Figure 2.

15. Federal Trade Commission 2002: vi.

16. Frank 2007: 1993.

17. Federal Trade Commission 2006. The data are for the fiscal year of 2005–06.

18. As this book goes to press, Congress is considering legislation that would regulate the use of "authorized" generic drugs.

19. McGuire 2007.

20. The price quotes are from Wal-Mart in Fairfax, Virginia, from February 2004 and December 2007.

21. A prescription is still needed from a physician to take advantage of free trial offers. The state of Massachusetts outlaws the use of free-trial coupons for prescription medication.

22. National Institute for Health Care Management 2002.

23. Centers for Medicare and Medicaid Services 2009: Tables 1, 11.

24. Insurance plans typically have three tiers for prescription drugs. The first tier includes the cheaper drugs such as generics with the lowest copay and fewest restrictions. The third tier includes the more expensive brand-name drugs. The copay for third tier drugs is higher and pre-authorization is often required. Some insurance companies have instituted a fourth tier with copay of $100 or more.

25. PhRMA 2007.

26. Pharmaceutical Industry Association of Puerto Rico Web site. www.piapr.com.

27. Government Accountability Office 2007: Table 2.

28. Government Accountability Office 2007; Stanglin 2007.

29. Government Accountability Office 2007: 3.

30. Melia 2007.

31. Bogdanich 2008a; Kaufman 2008a. The final count of documented death from contaminated heparin was 81.

32. Kaufman 2008b.

33. Reinberg 2008.

34. Harris 2008b; Gardner 2008. Contaminated heparin was identified in Australia, Canada, China, Denmark, France, Germany, Italy, Japan, the Netherlands, New Zealand, and the United States.

35. Bogdanich 2008b.

36. Harris and Bogdanich 2008.

37. Bogdanich 2008b.

38. Harris 2008b.

39. Frank 2007: 1993.

40. National Women's Health Network and Pharmedout.org 2007.

41. Freudenheim 2004.

42. Mukherjee et al. 2001; Topol 2004.

43. U.S. Food and Drug Administration 2004.

Chapter 5: Hospitals

1. Form newsletters: George Washington University Hospital, *Health News*, spring 2006, summer 2006, winter 2007; Georgetown University Hospital, *MyGeorgetownMD*, spring 2006, summer 2006; Sibley Memorial Hospital, *On Health*, fall 2005.

2. Pearlstein 2007.

3. Ibid.

4. HealthGrades 2008.

5. U.S. Census Bureau 2009b: Table 113. In comparison, 45,343 people died in motor vehicle accidents in 2005.

6. Zwillich 2006.

7. Nguyen 2009.

8. Klevens et al. 2007: 163; Sack 2007.

9. Sack 2007;

10. Siegel et al. 2006; Zwillich 2006.

11. Levine 2007a.

12. Mishori 2009.

13. Rein 2009.

14. Centers for Medicare and Medicaid Services 2007: 296–98. Medicare stopped paying for eight kinds of hospital-caused illnesses: surgery-site infections, ventilator-associated pneumonias, catheter-associated bloodstream infections, pressure ulcers, hospital falls, hospital-acquired pneumonia and certain bacterial infections, and "serious preventable event(s)." Serious preventable events include leaving an object in a patient's body during surgery, operation on the wrong body part or patient, air embolism as a result of surgery, and providing incompatible blood and blood products.

15. Golden and Jorgensen 2002.

16. Relman 2007: 31.

17. National health expenditures were $2,123 billion in 2006 according to data from Centers for Medicare and Medicaid Services (2007: Table 1). HCA Annual End-year Report of 2006 recorded $25 billion in revenues, which is 1.2 percent of national health expenditures.

18. U.S. Department of Justice 2000.

19. The first settlement in 2002 of $840 million in criminal fines and civil damages and penalties was for committing various forms of billing fraud. The second settlement in 2002 of $881 million related to filing false Medicare reports and paying doctors kickbacks.

20. Stolberg 2005.

21. Kirkpatrick 2005a; 2005b.

22. Silverman et al.1999. The study looked at per-person spending on Medicare patients admitted to a hospital in 1990. The study adjusted for patient characteristics, such as age, gender, and income, as well as for hospital characteristics, such as the number of hospital beds, number of physicians, and mortality rates.

23. Devereaux et al. 2002. A meta-analysis is a statistical review of a number of different studies. The authors reviewed 15 observational studies on mortality in for-profit hospitals in the United States between 1982 and 1995.

24. Tanne 2002.

25. Hartz et al. 1989; Bond et al. 1999.

26. Shahpoori and Smith 2005.

27. Centers for Medicare and Medicaid Services, 2009: Table 6. Data are from 2001 to 2009.

28. Centers for Medicare and Medicaid Services, 2009: Table 2. Data are for 2008.

29. American Hospital Association 2001: 3. The study found that 1 hour of emergency care required 1 hour of paperwork, while 1 hour of skilled nursing care required 30 minutes of paperwork.

30. McKay et al. 2008.

31. National Library of Medicine 2006.

32. Envision Hospital Group Corp. was formerly known as the Doctors Community Healthcare Corp.

33. Levine 2007b.

34. Nakamura 2007; Nakamura and Levine 2007.

Chapter 6: Laboratories

1. Keirans et al. 1996.

2. Other species of ticks carry Lyme disease as well, but according to tick biologist Dr. Roger Drummond, they do not attack humans.

3. Vredevoe, year unknown.

4. Montgomery et al. 2004; Ribeiro and Francischetti 2003; Das et al. 2001.

5. EUCALB 2007; Kuthejlova et al. 2001; Ribeiro and Francischetti 2003.

6. Drummond 2000: 14.

7. Seed ticks are less likely to carry diseases because they have not had their first blood meal. Once they become nymphs and feed on animals that are more likely to be infected with diseases, they are more likely to

transmit diseases than adult ticks. Nymphs are also far more common than adult ticks.

8. Bureau of Economic Analysis: "Personal consumption expenditures by product type." Underlying detail table, Table 2.4.5U. Data are for "medical laboratories" in 2008. Bureau of Labor Statistics: Employees on nonfarm payrolls by detailed industry. Medical and diagnostic laboratories. Establishment data. Annual employment for 2008.

9. Quest Diagnostics, Annual Report 2008, January 26, 2009.

10. "Company history" at www.questdiagnostics.com;

11. Laboratory Corporation of America, Annual Report 2008, February 12, 2009.

12. Quest Diagnostics, Explanation of benefits statement, May 2006.

13. My diary, description of my trip to Quest Diagnostic patient service center in downtown Washington DC, February 6, 2005.

14. ELISA stands for Enzyme Linked Immunosorbent Assay. It is an antibody test that measures the level of antibodies for a specific antigen, here the bacteria that causes Lyme disease.

15. Tugwell et al. 1997; Depietropaolo et al. 2005.

16. Stricker 2006.

17. Luger and Krauss 1990; Bakken et al. 1992.

18. Poon et al. 2004. The survey asked physicians to report delays in reviewing test results during the previous two months.

19. Casalino et al. 2009.

20. In states that require patients to obtain a requisition from their doctor for diagnostic tests, laboratories can circumvent the law by hiring doctors directly to sign off on the lab order form without seeing the patient.

21. QuestDirect closed down in 2006.

22. Tarkan 2002.

23. Ibid.

24. Health insurance companies buy access to patient records compiled by diagnostics laboratories, and therefore may gain access to test results.

25. American College of Physicians 1997.

Chapter 7: Lyme Disease

1. Weintraub 2008: 222.

2. Burgdorfer et al. 1982.

3. Marshall et al. 1994.

4. Dr. Oliver, a biologist at Georgia Southern University, mated the *I. dommini* and the *I. scapularis*, proving the two ticks were the same species.

5. Drummond 2000: 32.

6. Centers for Disease Control and Prevention 2009b.

7. Centers for Disease Control and Prevention 2004. The CDC has adopted a very strict definition of Lyme disease for surveillance purposes, which requires patients to have erythema migrans rash with known tick exposure (e.g., a tick bite); or if no bull's-eye rash is present, that at least one late manifestation exists along with two positive Lyme tests. According to the CDC's surveillance guidelines, a bull's-eye rash does not occur in 20–40 percent of all patients with Lyme disease (CDC 2008).

8. Lyme Disease Association, About Lyme Disease Web site, www .lymediseaseassociation.org/CasesLyme.html.

9. Tugwell et al. 1997; Depietropaolo et al. 2005.

10. Stricker 2006.

11. Porcella and Schwan 2001.

12. Casjens et al. 2000.

13. Brorson and Brorson 1997.

14. Embers et al. 2004.

15. Klempner et al. 2001: 85.

16. Fallon et al. 2008.

17. Krupp et al. 2003.

18. Wormser et al. 2006: 1094.

19. Wormser et al. 2006: 1094, 1120.

20. Cameron et al. 2004.

21. Connecticut Attorney General's Office 2008.

22. Anderson 2006.

23. Nery 2006.

24. Wormser et al. 2006: 1119.

25. Straubinger et al. 1998: 874.

26. Hodzic et al. 2008.

27. A 2005 study (Ruzic-Sabljic et al. 2005) found Lyme bacteria in the skin of three patients with the European strain of Lyme borrelia (*B. afzelii*) three months after completion of antibiotic therapy.

Chapter 8: Health Care Reform

1. Relman 2007: 64.

2. Author's own calculation based on the assumption that administrative cost of private health care plans is 17 percent, the mid-point of the range of estimates provided by Relman 2007; Commonwealth Fund 2008: 13.

3. UnitedHealth Group Web site: News Room, "UnitedHealth Group reports third quarter results," News release, October 16, 2008: 9.

4. Freed 2006.

5. Forelle and Bandler 2006.

6. Forelle and Maramont 2006.

7. U.S. Securities and Exchange Commission 2007.

8. National Health Care Anti-Fraud Association 2008.

9. Federal Bureau of Investigation 2008.

10. Girion 2008a.

11. Girion 2007.

12. Ornstein 2002.

13. Organisation for Economic Co-Operation and Development 2009.

14. Commonwealth Fund 2008: 19.

15. Nolte and McKee 2008.

16. U.S. Census Bureau 2009a: Table 7.

17. Henry J. Kaiser Family Foundation 2009b: Exhibit 1.1.

18. Relman 2007: 64. Administrative costs of Medicare are 12–33 percent of those of private insurance companies.

19. Longman 2007.

20. Mayo 2006.

21. Asch et al. 2004: 942.

22. Commonwealth Fund 2008: 20.

23. Relman 2007: 113.

24. Centers for Medicare and Medicaid Services 2009: Table 1.

Epilogue

1. Henry J. Kaiser Family Foundation 2009c.

2. Nagourney and Sussman 2009; *Washington Post* 2009.

3. Henry J. Kaiser Family Foundation 2009c.

4. Keyhani and Federman 2009.

5. Infectious Diseases Society of America Web site: http://webcast.you-niversity.com/idsaArchives/.

Index

About the Author

HELENE JORGENSEN is a senior research associate with the Center for Economic and Policy Research. She received her PhD in economics from American University, served as an advisor to the U.S. Census Bureau Advisory Committee on the Decennial Census, and chaired the Bureau of Labor Statistics Labor Research Advisory Committee. She previously worked at the AFL-CIO. She now serves as the moderator of the Washington DC Online Lyme Support Group (http://health.groups.yahoo.com/group/DCLyme).

Currently Jorgensen lives in Washington DC with her husband and two adopted dogs. She volunteers at the Washington Humane Society training pit bulls and is still recovering from neurological Lyme disease.

Other Books from PoliPointPress

The Blue Pages: A Directory of Companies Rated by Their Politics and Practices, 2nd edition

Helps consumers match their buying decisions with their political values by listing the political contributions and business practices of over 1,000 companies. $12.95, PAPERBACK.

Sasha Abramsky, *Breadline USA: The Hidden Scandal of American Hunger and How to Fix It*

Treats the increasing food insecurity crisis in America not only as a matter of failed policies, but also as an issue of real human suffering. $23.95, CLOTH.

Rose Aguilar, *Red Highways: A Liberal's Journey into the Heartland*

Challenges red state stereotypes to reveal new strategies for progressives. $15.95, PAPERBACK.

Dean Baker, *Plunder and Blunder: The Rise and Fall of the Bubble Economy*

Chronicles the growth and collapse of the stock and housing bubbles and explains how policy blunders and greed led to the catastrophic—but completely predictable—market meltdowns. $15.95, PAPERBACK.

Jeff Cohen, *Cable News Confidential: My Misadventures in Corporate Media*

Offers a fast-paced romp through the three major cable news channels—Fox CNN, and MSNBC—and delivers a serious message about their failure to cover the most urgent issues of the day. $14.95, PAPERBACK.

Marjorie Cohn, *Cowboy Republic: Six Ways the Bush Gang Has Defied the Law*

Shows how the executive branch under President Bush systematically defied the law instead of enforcing it. $14.95, PAPERBACK.

Marjorie Cohn and Kathleen Gilberd, *Rules of Disengagement: The Politics and Honor of Military Dissent*

Examines what U.S. military men and women have done—and what their families and others can do—to resist illegal wars, as well as military racism, sexual harassment, and denial of proper medical care. $14.95, PAPERBACK.

Joe Conason, *The Raw Deal: How the Bush Republicans Plan to Destroy Social Security and the Legacy of the New Deal*

Reveals the well-financed and determined effort to undo the Social Security Act and other New Deal programs. $11.00, PAPERBACK.

Kevin Danaher, Shannon Biggs, and Jason Mark, *Building the Green Economy: Success Stories from the Grassroots*

Shows how community groups, families, and individual citizens have protected their food and water, cleaned up their neighborhoods, and strengthened their local economies. $16.00, PAPERBACK.

Kevin Danaher and Alisa Gravitz, *The Green Festival Reader: Fresh Ideas from Agents of Change*

Collects the best ideas and commentary from some of the most forward green thinkers of our time. $15.95, PAPERBACK.

Reese Erlich, *Dateline Havana: The Real Story of U.S. Policy and the Future of Cuba*

Explores Cuba's strained relationship with the United States, the island nation's evolving culture and politics, and prospects for U.S.–Cuba policy with the departure of Fidel Castro. $22.95, HARDCOVER.

Reese Erlich, *The Iran Agenda: The Real Story of U.S. Policy and the Middle East Crisis*

Explores the turbulent recent history between the two countries and how it has led to a showdown over nuclear technology. $14.95, PAPERBACK.

Todd Farley, *Making the Grades: My Misadventures in the Standardized Testing Industry*

Exposes the folly of many large-scale educational assessments through an alternately edifying and hilarious first-hand account of life in the testing business. $16.95, PAPERBACK.

Steven Hill, *10 Steps to Repair American Democracy*

Identifies the key problems with American democracy, especially election practices, and proposes ten specific reforms to reinvigorate it. $11.00, PAPERBACK.

Jim Hunt, *They Said What? Astonishing Quotes on American Power, Democracy, and Dissent*

Covering everything from squashing domestic dissent to stymieing equal representation, these quotes remind progressives exactly what they're up against. $12.95, PAPERBACK.

Michael Huttner and Jason Salzman, *50 Ways You Can Help Obama Change America*

Describes actions citizens can take to clean up the mess from the last administration, enact Obama's core campaign promises, and move the country forward. $12.95, PAPERBACK.

Markos Kounalakis and Peter Laufer, *Hope Is a Tattered Flag: Voices of Reason and Change for the Post-Bush Era*

Gathers together the most listened-to politicos and pundits, activists and thinkers, to answer the question: what happens after Bush leaves office? $29.95, HARD-COVER; $16.95 PAPERBACK.

Yvonne Latty, *In Conflict: Iraq War Veterans Speak Out on Duty, Loss, and the Fight to Stay Alive*

Features the unheard voices, extraordinary experiences, and personal photographs of a broad mix of Iraq War veterans, including Congressman Patrick Murphy, Tammy Duckworth, Kelly Daugherty, and Camilo Mejia. $24.00, HARDCOVER.

Phillip Longman, *Best Care Anywhere: Why VA Health Care Is Better Than Yours*

Shows how the turnaround at the long-maligned VA hospitals provides a blueprint for salvaging America's expensive but troubled health care system. $14.95, PAPERBACK.

Phillip Longman and Ray Boshara, *The Next Progressive Era*

Provides a blueprint for a re-empowered progressive movement and describes its implications for families, work, health, food, and savings. $22.95, HARDCOVER.

Marcia and Thomas Mitchell, *The Spy Who Tried to Stop a War: Katharine Gun and the Secret Plot to Sanction the Iraq Invasion*

Describes a covert operation to secure UN authorization for the Iraq war and the furor that erupted when a young British spy leaked it. $23.95, HARDCOVER.

Susan Mulcahy, ed., *Why I'm a Democrat*

Explores the values and passions that make a diverse group of Americans proud to be Democrats. $14.95, PAPERBACK.

David Neiwert, *The Eliminationists: How Hate Talk Radicalized the American Right*

Argues that the conservative movement's alliances with far-right extremists have not only pushed the movement's agenda to the right, but also have become a malignant influence increasingly reflected in political discourse. $16.95, PAPERBACK.

Christine Pelosi, *Campaign Boot Camp: Basic Training for Future Leaders*

Offers a seven-step guide for successful campaigns and causes at all levels of government. $15.95, PAPERBACK.

William Rivers Pitt, *House of Ill Repute: Reflections on War, Lies, and America's Ravaged Reputation*

Skewers the Bush Administration for its reckless invasions, warrantless wiretaps, lethally incompetent response to Hurricane Katrina, and other scandals and blunders. $16.00, PAPERBACK.

Sarah Posner, *God's Profits: Faith, Fraud, and the Republican Crusade for Values Voters*

Examines corrupt televangelists' ties to the Republican Party and unprecedented access to the Bush White House. $19.95, HARDCOVER.

Nomi Prins, *Jacked: How "Conservatives" Are Picking Your Pocket — Whether You Voted for Them or Not*

Describes how the "conservative" agenda has affected your wallet, skewed national priorities, and diminished America—but not the American spirit. $12.00, PAPERBACK.

Cliff Schecter, *The Real McCain: Why Conservatives Don't Trust Him— and Why Independents Shouldn't*

Explores the gap between the public persona of John McCain and the reality of this would-be president. $14.95, HARDCOVER.

Norman Solomon, *Made Love, Got War: Close Encounters with America's Warfare State*

Traces five decades of American militarism and the media's all-too-frequent failure to challenge it. $24.95, HARDCOVER.

John Sperling et al., *The Great Divide: Retro vs. Metro America*

Explains how and why our nation is so bitterly divided into what the authors call Retro and Metro America. $19.95, PAPERBACK.

Daniel Weintraub, *Party of One: Arnold Schwarzenegger and the Rise of the Independent Voter*

Explains how Schwarzenegger found favor with independent voters, whose support has been critical to his success, and suggests that his bipartisan approach represents the future of American politics. $19.95, HARDCOVER.

Curtis White, *The Barbaric Heart: Faith, Money, and the Crisis of Nature*

Argues that the solution to the present environmental crisis may come from an unexpected quarter: the arts, religion, and the realm of the moral imagination. $16.95, PAPERBACK.

Curtis White, *The Spirit of Disobedience: Resisting the Charms of Fake Politics, Mindless Consumption, and the Culture of Total Work*

Debunks the notion that liberalism has no need for spirituality and describes a "middle way" through our red state/blue state political impasse. Includes three powerful interviews with John DeGraaf, James Howard Kunstler, and Michael Ableman. $24.00, HARDCOVER.

For more information, please visit www.p3books.com.

About This Book

This book is printed on Cascade Enviro100 Print paper. It contains 100 percent post-consumer fiber and is certified EcoLogo, Processed Chlorine Free, and FSC Recycled. For each ton used instead of virgin paper, we:

- Save the equivalent of 17 trees
- Reduce air emissions by 2,098 pounds
- Reduce solid waste by 1,081 pounds
- Reduce the water used by 10,196 gallons
- Reduce suspended particles in the water by 6.9 pounds.

This paper is manufactured using biogas energy, reducing natural gas consumption by 2,748 cubic feet per ton of paper produced.

The book's printer, Malloy Incorporated, works with paper mills that are environmentally responsible, that do not source fiber from endangered forests, and that are third-party certified. Malloy prints with soy- and vegetable-based inks, and over 98 percent of the solid material they discard is recycled. Their water emissions are entirely safe for disposal into their municipal sanitary sewer system, and they work with the Michigan Department of Environmental Quality to ensure that their air emissions meet all environmental standards.

The Michigan Department of Environmental Quality has recognized Malloy as a Great Printer for their compliance with environmental regulations, written environmental policy, pollution prevention efforts, and pledge to share best practices with other printers. Their county Department of Planning and Environment has designated them a Waste Knot Partner for their waste prevention and recycling programs.